Occupational Therapy and Chronic Fatigue Syndrome

Occupational Therapy and Chronic Fatigue Syndrome

DIANE L. COX PhD MSc DipCOT

Senior Lecturer in Occupational Therapy
South Bank University, London

Consulting Editor in Occupational Therapy
CLEPHANE HUME

W

WHURR PUBLISHERS
LONDON AND PHILADELPHIA

© 2000 Whurr Publishers
First published 2000 by
Whurr Publishers Ltd
19b Compton Terrace, London N1 2UN, England and
325 Chestnut Street, Philadelphia PA 19106, USA.

Reprinted 2004

British Library Cataloguing in Publication Data
A catalogue record for this book is available from the
British Library.

ISBN: 1 86156 155 5

Printed and bound in the UK by Athenaeum Press Ltd,
Gateshead, Tyne & Wear

Contents

Preface

Occupational Therapy and Chronic Fatigue Syndrome aims to encourage and assist students and clinicians in the understanding of chronic fatigue syndrome (CFS) and its management. It aims to provide the reader with an in-depth overview of the current information on aetiology, treatment and practical evidence-based management of CFS, with specific emphasis on occupational therapy intervention.

Working with people who have CFS involves all aspects of the occupational therapy process; many of the skills we gain in training and in other areas of clinical practice can be transferred to the management of CFS. The aim of this book is to demystify the illness and its management, and to show how a great deal can be done by the occupational therapist to help the patient towards recovery.

The first section begins with an introduction to the diagnostic criteria, aetiology, clinical features and prevalence and prognosis. This is followed by an overview of the history of CFS. Section Two discusses the clinical assessment and pharmacological management of CFS. Section Three discusses and explores the current treatment approaches in CFS and Section Four deals in depth with the service developed by the author and a specific occupational therapy approach to management. Section Five deals with research, measurement and future directions. Throughout the book, case vignettes and more in-depth case studies have been used to illustrate the syndrome and its management. There are a number of appendices providing additional information including examples of booklets, information sheets and useful addresses. The appendices are followed by a glossary of terms.

It is hoped that *Occupational Therapy and Chronic Fatigue Syndrome* will assist both students and clinicians who are new to CFS, by helping them use their professional skills to enable people with CFS to achieve an increase in activity levels and ultimately regain their ability to lead a productive life.

Acknowledgements

From conception to completion of this book there are many people to thank. If I have missed anyone, I offer my apologies. The book could not have been conceived without the contact with, and support of, the patient group over the last 10 years, to whom I am grateful.

I would like to thank specifically: Professor Leslie J. Findley, Consultant Neurologist, for his continuing support, encouragement and guidance; all members of the chronic fatique syndrome team past and present, in particular Sue Codd, Lindsey Barker and Charlie Leuchars for their support, their flexibility in being ready to try out new ideas and their influence; Professor Jeni Wilson-Barnett and Dr Alison Richardson, of King's College, London, my PhD supervisors, the work for which forms part of the book; my occupational therapy colleagues at South Bank University, who supported me through the final stages of completion; in particular, Judith Payling, who made extremely useful suggestions as regards the final presentation and content of the book; and finally to my family, friends and colleagues who put up with my moans, fears and anxieties over the years, especially Mark, thank you.

Introduction

The impetus for this book came from this author's work as a clinical occupational therapist with patients diagnosed as having chronic fatigue syndrome (CFS). However, the inspiration for the book came from the numerous enquiries received over the last nine years from occupational therapists, physiotherapists, nurses and general practitioners for advice and guidance on the management of people with CFS. In particular, the author was increasingly contacted by occupational therapists working with a wide range of caseloads and in varied settings such as: acute physical, mental health, paediatrics and social services. This book therefore aims to meet the need of occupational therapists for advice on management in this new and important area.

In the early 1990s the hospital in which the author worked was one of the few centres diagnosing and treating people with CFS (Cox and Findley, 1994). The development of the service within an acute NHS neurological sciences centre aimed to meet an empirical demand to diagnose and treat patients on an inpatient and or outpatient basis as required by clinical need (Cox and Findley, 1994, 1998; Cox 1998). Recently the Royal Colleges' Report (1996) stated that most people with CFS could be treated in primary care and that cognitive behaviour therapy (CBT) (Sharpe et al., 1996; Deale et al., 1997) and prescribed graded aerobic exercise (Fulcher and White, 1997) appeared to be promising approaches in outpatient management.

However, the report suggested that a minority of patients would require inpatient care. This would enable access to a multi-professional team; time for education into lifestyle management techniques; consolidation and reinforcement of information given; time for questioning and clinical assessment, evaluation and investigations (Royal Colleges, 1996; Cox and Findley, 1998). In certain instances, patients need a change in environment in order to break the dynamics that may be perpetuating the illness (Lloyd et al., 1993; Cox and Findley, 1998). Others have recognized the need for severely cognitively and or physically incapacitated patients to be admitted to hospital (Chalder, Butler and Wessely, 1996; Essame et al., 1998).

Occupational therapists work towards maximizing levels of independence and ability. In the treatment of CFS it is the task of the occupational therapist to work with each patient individually, facilitating lifestyle changes as required. The aim of occupational therapy is to help the person with CFS gain a better understanding of the illness and how to cope with it (Cox, 1999a). This would include talking through current abilities, routines and ways of coping. The occupational therapist would discuss the person's current lifestyle, and then offer the opportunity to look at ways of making adjustments so that, in time, the person is able to do more.

The occupational therapy lifestyle management programme is tailored to each individual's need and taken at each person's pace. This may mean that information is covered at different speeds and in different environments as an outpatient or, for some, as an inpatient. Written information is used to support the discussion about the various aspects of lifestyle management. Lifestyle management education does not represent a 'cure' for CFS. Neither is it prescriptive or inflexible. It is designed to help the sufferer learn methods of coping with the illness, feel more in control of the symptoms and increase his/her potential for recovery.

Section One:
Current Understanding of
Chronic Fatigue Syndrome

In the last 20 years there has been substantial debate and discussion surrounding chronic fatigue syndrome, which hitherto in the UK was given the title myalgic encephalomyelitis (Ramsey, 1978). In the absence of a complete understanding of the mechanisms behind this heterogeneous group of disorders, a number of very precise definitions for diagnosis (Holmes et al., 1988; Sharpe et al., 1991; Fukuda et al., 1994) have been developed for the purposes of research and clinical guidance. In addition, the Royal Colleges' Report (1996) although subject to criticism (*Lancet*, 1996), has stated categorically that these disorders pose significant morbidity, they need to be recognized and treatment programmes developed with an emphasis on primary care.

Chapter 1
What is Chronic Fatigue Syndrome?

Definition and Diagnostic Criteria

Historically, many chronic illnesses have been difficult to define. Specific causative agents are often unknown and diagnostic laboratory tests often have poor sensitivity and specificity (Holmes et al., 1988; Holmes, 1991). Hence, case definitions have been developed through the consensus of expert committees for such illnesses as rheumatoid arthritis, systemic lupus erythematosus and various psychiatric illnesses (Holmes, 1991).

Owing to the unknown aetiology of the illness, specific definition and diagnostic criteria for chronic fatigue syndrome (CFS) were essential to increase understanding, to aid study of the illness and to determine subgroups (Holmes, 1991). Laboratory tests in CFS have also been shown to contribute little to assessment, diagnosis and treatment because of insufficient sensitivity and explicitness (Vercoulen et al., 1994; Bates et al., 1995). Fulfilment of specific criteria would also ensure that other diagnoses such as fibromyalgia were not missed (Goldenberg et al., 1986).

The illness was originally defined in 1988 by a group of American clinicians and researchers working with CFS who met at the Center for Disease Control (CDC) in Atlanta, Georgia, USA (Holmes et al., 1988). Prior to the publication of this definition the illness in the USA had been known as chronic Epstein–Barr virus syndrome. However, doubt had been cast on the relationship between Epstein–Barr and the development of a fatigue state (Buchwald et al., 1987). A new name was therefore proposed, that of CFS (Holmes et al., 1988). CFS described the most noticeable characteristic of the syndrome without implying a causal relationship. As the syndrome had no diagnostic test, the working definition proposed was based on signs and symptoms only (see Figure 1.1). To be defined as CFS a case had to fulfil major criteria 1 and 2, and a certain number of minor criteria: six or more of the 11 symptom criteria and two or more of the three physical criteria; or eight or more of the 11 symptom criteria (Holmes et al., 1988) as cited in Figure 1.1.

MAJOR CRITERIA
1.   New onset of persistent or relapsing, debilitating fatigue or easy fatigability in a person who has no previous history of similar symptoms, that does not resolve with bedrest, and that is severe enough to reduce or impair average daily activity below 50% of the patient's premorbid activity level for a period of at least six months.
2.   Other clinical conditions that may produce similar symptoms must be excluded by thorough evaluation, based on history, physical examination and appropriate laboratory findings. These include: malignancy, autoimmune disease; localized infection; chronic or subacute bacterial disease; fungal disease and parasitic disease; chronic psychiatric disease; chronic inflammatory disease; neuromuscular disease; endocrine disease; drug dependency or abuse; side effects of a chronic medication or other toxic agent; or other known or defined pulmonary, cardiac, gastrointestinal, hepatic, renal or haematological disease.

If any results of tests are abnormal the physician should search for other conditions that may cause such a result. If no such conditions are detected by reasonable evaluation, the criterion is satisfied.

MINOR CRITERIA
Symptom Criteria
To fulfil a symptom criteria, a symptom must have begun at or after the time of onset of increased fatigability, and must have persisted, or recurred, over a period of at least six months. Symptoms include:
1.   Mild fever
2.   Sore throat
3.   Painful lymph nodes in the anterior, or posterior cervical, or axillary distribution
4.   Unexplained generalized muscle weakness
5.   Muscle discomfort or myalgia
6.   Prolonged (24 hours or greater) generalized fatigue after levels of exercise that would have been easily tolerated in the patient's premorbid state
7.   Generalized headaches
8.   Migratory arthralgia without joint swelling or redness
9.   Neuropsychologic complaints
10. Sleep disturbance (hypersomnia or insomnia)
11. Description of the main symptom complex as initially developing over a few hours or days

Physical Criteria
Physical criteria must be documented by a physician on at least two occasions, at least 1 month apart.
1.   Low grade fever
2.   Nonexudative pharyngitis
3.   Palpable or tender anterior or posterior cervical or axillary lymph nodes

Source: Holmes et al. (1988)

Figure 1.1 1988 CDC criteria for CFS.

The definition became known as the 1988 CDC criteria. However, these proved difficult to use in practice (Kormaroff and Geiger, 1989). It was found that the definition was frequently modified owing to difficulty in interpreting the criteria and compliance with them (Straus, 1992). The inconsistency in interpretation and application of the CDC definition was confirmed by Schluederberg and colleagues (1992). An Australian definition published by Lloyd and colleagues (1988) was also reported to be unsatisfactory in practice and was not widely accepted (Sharpe et al., 1991).

In an attempt to resolve difficulties encountered in using the 1988 CDC criteria (Holmes et al., 1988), a group of UK clinicians and scientists who were involved in CFS research met in Oxford, UK, to redefine CFS (Sharpe et al., 1991). It was agreed that CFS was the best name, as it was descriptive and free from unproven aetiological implications. The main differences between the definitions were the statement that illness should not be lifelong, and certain exclusions of schizophrenia, manic depressive illness, substance abuse, eating disorder or organic brain disorder were cited. In addition, a subtype of CFS was defined and named post infectious fatigue syndrome (PIFS) (Sharpe et al., 1991). PIFS was defined as fatigue following an infection, or associated with a current infection and the infection should be corroborated by laboratory evidence. However, this definition did not gain wide recognition.

The 1988 CDC criteria were also criticized for not explicitly defining certain terms and not specifying the duration and quality of bedrest and the rigour of neurologic and psychiatric evaluations (Armon and Kurland, 1991). As exclusion of other illness was a major criterion of CFS, in practice confusion centred on the role of depression (Bell, 1992). The UK definition (Sharpe et al., 1991) stated that depressive illness, anxiety and hyperventilation syndrome were not necessarily reasons for exclusion.

An international group of clinicians, scientists and researchers therefore met at the CDC to propose a conceptual framework to enable an integrated and comprehensive approach to the study of CFS (Fukuda et al., 1994). This definition has become the most accepted. It suggests three subdivisions: CFS, post viral fatigue syndrome and idiopathic chronic fatigue. All the case definitions (Holmes et al., 1988; Lloyd et al., 1988; Sharpe et al., 1991; Fukuda et al., 1994) require considerable morbidity from new fatigue in excess of six months with all other recognized causes of fatigue having been excluded by history, observation and clinical assessment. To comply with the 1994 CDC criteria the patient must fulfil both major points, 1 and 2, and present with four or more of the symptoms listed in point 3 shown in Figure 1.2 (Fukuda et al., 1994, pp. 954–956).

(1) New onset of self-reported persistent or relapsing, debilitating fatigue in a person who has no previous history of similar symptoms, that has lasted for six months or longer, is disabling and affects physical and mental functioning and:
   (a) is characterized by fatigue as the principal symptom;
   (b) is of new or definite onset (has not been lifelong);
   (c) is not the result of ongoing exertion;
   (d) is not substantially alleviated by rest;
   (e) results in substantial reduction in previous levels of occupation, educational, social or personal activities.
(2) Other clinical conditions that may produce similar symptoms, including preexisting psychiatric diseases, must be excluded by thorough evaluation, based on history, physical examination and appropriate laboratory findings. These conditions will include:
   (a) any active medical condition;
   (b) any previously diagnosed medical condition whose continued activity may explain the illness, such as previously treated malignancies and unresolved cases of hepatitis B or C infection;
   (c) any past or current diagnosis of major depressive disorder, including bipolar affective disorder, schizophrenia, delusional disorders, dementia, anorexia nervosa or bulimia nervosa;
   (d) alcohol or substance abuse within two years;
   (e) severe obesity.
(3) Four or more of the following symptoms must be concurrently present for six or more months:
   (a) impaired concentration or memory;
   (b) sore throat;
   (c) tender cervical or axillary lymph nodes;
   (d) muscle pain;
   (e) multi-joint pain without joint swelling or redness;
   (f) headaches of a new type, pattern or severity;
   (g) unrefreshing sleep;
   (h) post-exertional malaise lasting more than 24 hours.

To meet the criteria for post viral fatigue syndrome (PVFS) patients must:

(1) fulfil the criteria for CFS as defined above;
(2) have definite evidence of infection at onset or presentation (a patient's self-report is unlikely to be sufficiently reliable) and should fulfil the following criteria:
   (a) the syndrome is present for a minimum of six months after onset of infection;
   (b) the infection has been corroborated by laboratory evidence.

If the criteria for CFS or PVFS are not met, the fatigue is lifelong and no other cause for the fatigue is identified, a classification of *idiopathic chronic fatigue* would be given.

Source: Fukuda et al. (1994)

Figure 1.2 1994 CDC criteria for CFS.

Aetiology

There is no one theory on the actual cause of CFS. Currently it is thought that different causes or triggers start the illness but result in the same outcome of CFS (Wessely et al., 1989; Surawy et al., 1995). Many researchers have explored a number of possible causative agents, which include:

- infection;
- central nervous system abnormalities;
- chronic immune activation;
- neuromuscular factors;
- psychiatric factors.

Infection

Patients frequently cite an acute 'infection' or 'viral' illness at onset which may not be confirmed on laboratory testing (Lloyd et al., 1990a; Wessely et al., 1995). They often state that their chronic illness 'all started with that virus that never went away' (Kormaroff and Buchwald, 1998, p. 3). Two primary care studies have been carried out in the UK with the aim of determining a relationship between viral illness and the onset of chronic fatigue six months later (Cope et al., 1994; Wessely et al., 1995). In the large cohort study carried out by Wessely and colleagues (1995) they were unable to show any role for common viral infections as aetiological factors. In contrast, Cope and colleagues (1994) found that, at six months following GP-reported acute viral infections, 17.5% of patients remained chronically fatigued.

In the 1980s in the UK, persistent enteroviral infection, in particular Coxsackie B viruses, were implicated in CFS (Calder et al., 1987; Dowsett et al., 1990), and the VP-1 antigen was reported as a possible diagnostic marker (Yousef et al., 1988). However, later investigation did not confirm these findings (Halpin and Wessely, 1989; Lynch and Seth, 1989; Gow et al., 1994; Joyce and Wessely, 1996). In the USA, infective mononucleosis (Epstein–Barr virus) was suggested as a causative factor (Holmes et al., 1988). Doubt was cast on the conclusive evidence of Epstein–Barr virus as the prime cause of CFS, and the possible value of Epstein–Barr virus antibody testing as a diagnostic marker (Kormaroff and Geiger, 1988) following investigation in a general medical practice (Buchwald et al., 1987) and university health centre (Matthews et al., 1991). However, a more recent study in the UK elucidated some evidence of the probable existence of a fatigue syndrome following glandular fever, although not necessarily fulfilling the criteria for CFS (White et al., 1995).

Post-infectious fatigue has been noted after brucellosis, influenza, Epstein–Barr virus, Lyme disease and enterovirus (Imboden et al., 1961; White et al., 1995; Salit, 1997). However, the persistence of such viruses has been shown not to play a part in the pathogenesis of CFS (Gow et al., 1994; Swanink et al., 1995) and to date no evidence of a single infecting agent has been found (Salit, 1997). Viral infection in the community is common though, and the possibility of chance associations between viral infection and the onset of fatigue cannot be excluded (Wessely, 1995b).

Neuromuscular Factors

Neurophysiological explanations have been explored, as most patients complain of profound fatigue and myalgia after exertion, predominantly affecting the muscles (Bearn and Wessely, 1994). Mitochondrial abnormalities have been reported (Behan et al., 1991), and a greater subjective sensation of fatigue and a difficulty in reaching maximal effort has been shown in patients with CFS (Riley et al., 1990; Lloyd et al., 1991). However, this work excluded a simple neuromuscular problem as a credible explanation for CFS (David et al., 1988) and started to pose questions about higher cortical mechanisms (above the level of the motor cortex) and the connection between motor control and feedback (Lloyd et al., 1991).

Central Nervous System

Patients with CFS often complain of symptoms that suggest central nervous system (CNS) involvement. These include cognitive symptoms such as difficulty with concentration, attention and memory, and other symptoms such as photophobia, paresthesia, vertigo and imbalance and headache (Kormaroff and Buchwald, 1998).

Evidence now suggests that changes in the neurobiological mechanisms underlying the stress response at, or above, the level of the hypothalamus, in particular the hypothalamic–pituitary–adrenal axis (HPA), may be relevant to the pathophysiology of CFS (Demitrack et al., 1991; Cleare et al., 1995). Stress-induced activation of the HPA involves activation of 5-hydroxytryptamine (5-HT) neurones (Bearn and Wessely, 1994) and resultant neuroendocrine dysfunction can cause hypocortisolism and upregulation of 5-HT receptors in the hypothalamus (Demitrack et al., 1991; Cleare et al., 1995). As the HPA strongly influences the autonomic nervous system, changes to this function could induce signs of physiological and behavioural arousal, including sympathetic nervous system activation and hyper-responsiveness to sensory stimuli (Demitrack et al., 1991). This may be an explanation as to why patients complain of such diverse symptoms as:

- mood changes;
- nausea;
- dizziness;
- tinnitus;
- temperature control problems;
- sleep disturbance;
- anxiety;
- breathing dysfunction.

The 5-HT neurones are involved in particular with the control of sleep, appetite and mood (Cleare et al., 1995). Different and separable effects on the HPA axis and 5-HT function have been observed in CFS and depression (Cleare et al., 1995). This is an important observation, as some observers have doubted that there is any biological basis for CFS, and have postulated that it represents some form of depression, many patients being told 'it's all in your head' or 'you're just depressed' (Kormoroff and Buchwald, 1998). Interestingly, comparable HPA changes have been found in CFS and fibromyalgia, possibly indicating some degree of commonality between the syndromes (Moldofsky, 1995). Buchwald and Garrity (1994) found that demographic and clinical factors, and health beliefs and locus of control did not clearly distinguish patients with CFS and fibromyalgia.

However, a recent study failed to replicate the HPA changes in CFS patients (Young et al., 1998). A possible reason for failure to replicate previous findings was the type of patient group and their duration of symptoms. In the study by Young and colleagues (1998) patients were referred from primary care with a mean duration of symptoms of 2.5 years whereas, in previous studies, patients were referred from secondary and tertiary care (Demitrack et al., 1991; Cleare et al., 1995), and had a mean duration of symptoms of 7.2 years (Demitrack et al., 1991). This may indicate that HPA involvement is dependent on the chronicity of the illness and is therefore a consequence of the illness rather than a cause.

Some specific diagnostic studies of the CNS have found abnormalities in patients with CFS using techniques such as magnetic resonance imaging (MRI), single-photon emission computed tomography (SPECT) (Kormaroff and Buchwald, 1998) and sensory and cognitive event-related potentials (ERPs) (Prasher et al., 1990). As yet, though, there has been no identifiable pattern to the abnormalities seen through testing, for any of these to be considered as a diagnostic test. There has also been little consistency in the abnormal findings reported between the tests (Cope and David, 1996). In addition, the neuroimaging abnormalities have not yet been correlated with clinical findings in CFS (Bearn and Wessely, 1994; Cope and David,

1996), and therefore the role of CNS abnormalities seen in the pathophysiology of CFS is yet to be determined (Kormaroff and Buchwald, 1998).

The role of the CNS has been further explored through a number of studies on sleep disorder. Most patients with CFS complain of difficulty getting off to sleep, sleeping lightly and being unrefreshed on waking (Moldofsky, 1995). Morriss and colleagues (1993) postulated that the sleep disorder associated with the illness could be important in the aetiology of CFS, as the effects of sleep loss on performance of patients with sleep disorders were similar to the complaints of patients with CFS which include:

- increased subjective effort on exertion and slower subsequent recovery;
- reduced vigilance;
          attention span;
          cognitive performance.
(Morriss et al., 1993)

However, in a later study (Morriss et al., 1997) the group could find little evidence that disrupted sleep is associated with the onset of CFS. Instead, waking at night was often associated with pain and feeling hot or cold. They proposed that disrupted sleep was therefore:

> ...linked to physiological and psychological mechanisms involved with the production of myalgia or abnormal sensitivity to pain or temperature disturbance rather than physical or mental fatigue. (p. 605)

Sharpley and colleagues (1997) confirmed this conclusion by stating that:

> ...sleep abnormalities are merely an epiphenomenon. If patients have sought to overcome their fatigue by spending longer in bed at night and sleeping during the day, the observed sleep inefficiency could be simply a consequence of this behaviour. (p. 595)

Therefore abnormalities of sleep do not appear to be of major importance in the aetiology of CFS, but rather a consequence of the illness which can worsen over time (Morriss et al., 1997; Sharpley et al., 1997).

Further evidence as to the involvement of CNS dysfunction in CFS has been highlighted by the studies that have considered the cognitive impairment expressed by the majority of patients (Marshall et al., 1997; Kormaroff and Buchwald, 1998). DeLuca and colleagues (1993) concluded that selective impairment in information processing, in particular auditory material, could be the root of other cognitive complaints made by patients with CFS and confirmed this finding in a later study (DeLuca et al., 1995). It has been postulated that impaired information-processing ability in patients with CFS may be due to changes in cerebral white matter (DeLuca et al., 1995). However, a quantitative summary of the most rigorous MRI studies has shown no significant increase in white-matter lesions in CFS (Cope and David, 1996).

Psychiatric Factors

Joyce et al. (1996) identified that cognitive dysfunction was related to:

> ...reduced attentional capacity which results in impaired performance on effortful tasks requiring planned or self-ordered generation of responses from memory. (p. 495)

They also showed that there was little evidence that the deficits seen in CFS reflected a depressive illness. McDonald and colleagues (McDonald, Cope and David, 1993) also noted that the cognitive impairment found could not be explained by the presence of depression amongst patients with CFS. However the nature of the information-processing deficit is shown to be undistinguished from depression and appears to be a common deficit in both disorders (DeLuca et al., 1995; Marshall et al., 1997). In an effortful cognitive recall task on written information, slight evidence that CFS patients (whether depressed or not) were impaired has been noted (Wearden and Appleby, 1997).

DeLuca and colleagues (1997) subsequently concurred with McDonald and colleagues (1993) that the impaired cognition could not be explained solely by the presence of a psychiatric condition (primarily major depression) and that cognitive dysfunction was not induced by depression. In addition, they found that cognitive functioning was worse in CFS without a co-morbid psychiatric condition (DeLuca et al., 1997). In a later study (Christodoulou et al., 1998), it was also found that cognitive impairment was related to functional disability that could not be explained on the basis of psychiatric factors. These results, although they did not assist in confirming the aetiology of CFS, have implications for treatment. DeLuca and colleagues (1997) suggested that:

> ...patients with CFS with psychiatric complications may benefit more from psychotherapy in conjunction with psychopharmacological interventions. By contrast, patients without psychiatric co-morbidity may benefit more from a psycho-educational approach to symptom management or cognitive rehabilitation. (p. 154)

Marshall and colleagues (1997) suggested that the depression seen in CFS was a reaction to the illness and usually developed well after the onset of CFS and therefore might be considered a 'reactive depression' rather than major depression, thus adding weight to the conclusion that previous psychiatric disorder does not cause CFS but is a consequence of the disorder (Hickie et al., 1990). It would appear that primary major depression does not account for the cognitive difficulties found in CFS patients (Marshall et al., 1997).

Many patients with CFS do not suffer from mood, anxiety or somatization disorders (Kormaroff and Buchwald, 1998). However, one explanation for the possible link between CFS and psychiatric disorder sometimes seen as a consequence of or prior to the illness is that it may be due to some common neurobiological dysfunction rather than misdiagnosed cases of depression and anxiety (Joyce and Wessely, 1996; Cleare, 1997). The estimated prevalence of pre-morbid lifetime total psychiatric disorder in CFS has been put at 24% and major depression at 12.5% (Hickie et al., 1990).

The argument as to whether the cognitive deficits and/or psychiatric factors are due to a psychological consequence or aetiology in CFS is not conclusive. However, evidence of a consistent pattern of neuropsychological impairment is available including slower reaction times and information processing, and poorer performance on complex attentional and memory tasks (Moss-Morris et al., 1996; DeLuca et al., 1997).

Immune Dysfunction

Considerable attention has been given to the possible role of immune dysfunction in CFS (Wessely, 1995a). Various abnormalities have been suggested, but only a few have been consistently reported: elevated levels of immune complexes (IgG levels); increased numbers of CD8+ cytotoxic T cells; and depressed function of natural killer lymphocytes (Bates et al., 1995; Komaroff and Buchwald, 1998). These abnormalities may be evidence of ongoing activation of the immune system in CFS (Bates et al., 1995). However, the theory that a state of immune activation could disrupt neurotransmitter function and result in the symptoms of CFS remains unproven (Bearn and Wessely, 1994; Kormaroff and Buchwald, 1998). It also remains to be seen whether the immune abnormalities observed distinguish patients with CFS from other illnesses that could mimic CFS clinically, such as systemic lupus erythematosus (Buchwald and Kormaroff, 1991).

In conclusion, despite all the studies discussed, as yet there is no definitive cause for CFS. All reports appear to point towards CNS mechanisms but it is unclear whether they are primary or secondary to the illness and decreased physical activity. All agree that well-designed rigorous studies with appropriate statistical power are required. Current theory appears to suggest that the cause is multi-factorial, and that a combination of infective, physiological and psychological factors that creates dysfunction within the CNS is involved (Wessely, 1995b; Salit, 1997).

Clinical Features and Presentation

In 1994 Leitch described CFS as 'a complex amalgam of social, cultural, psychological and somatic factors' (p. 501). He makes the point that these factors and their interactions need to be addressed if a satisfactory outcome is to be possible (Leitch, 1994).

Clinical Features

From clinical experience, the commonest presentation seems to occur as a result of chronic stressors in a vulnerable individual (Cox and Findley, 1998). The other primary contributing factor is the report of a 'flu-like' illness at the onset (Salit, 1997; Kormaroff and Buchwald, 1998). The main complaint is persistent fatigue that differs from normal tiredness. The extreme fatigue affects both mental and physical capacity, reducing a person's activity ability substantially below his/her previous level of functioning (Joyce and Wessely, 1996; Cox, 1998). It is accompanied by a range of other unpleasant symptoms, such as:

- muscle and/ or joint pain;
- daily headache;
- recurrent sore throats;
- fluctuations in mood;
- intolerance of alcohol;
- cognitive processing difficulties which result in poor concentration and memory problems;
- autonomic changes such as temperature control problems, night sweats, digestive changes and palpitations (Hickie et al., 1995; Kormaroff and Buchwald, 1998; Cox, 1998).

A 'triangle of pain' from the posterior base of the skull to below the scapulae is often described, predominantly affecting the upper part of the trapezius (Cox, 1998).

Problems with sleep are common, and include sleeping longer than normal often at the beginning of the illness, and having difficulty getting off to sleep and waking frequently as the illness progresses (Morriss et al., 1993; Moldofsky, 1995). Whatever the problem, the sleep is seldom refreshing (Sharpe et al., 1997). The overall symptoms vary in degree in each individual (Behan and Behan, 1988) and are exacerbated by minimal exertion, unexplained by conventional biomedical diagnosis (Sharpe et al., 1997).

The degree of dysfunction can vary from mild to very severe (Behan and Behan, 1988). Mild is the level where patients are still mobile for short distances, able to carry out some outdoor activities and continue to work part time. Very severe is assessed to be when the patient is totally dependent on the support of others and predominantly in bed (Cox and Findley, 1998). In more severely affected individuals late-stage anxiety is often seen (Cox, 1998).

Presentation

Certain factors are thought to predispose, precipitate (trigger) and perpetuate the illness and what precipitates or causes CFS may not necessarily perpetuate it (Surawy et al., 1995). The perpetuators are often the effects of inactivity, inconsistent activity, illness beliefs and fears about symptoms and symptom focusing (Joyce and Wessely, 1996; Sharpe et al., 1996).

From experience the predisposing factors to the illness appear to be prolonged high striving and achievement, i.e. the person has a tendency to overwork, sets high standards and tends not to stop for illness (Surawy et al., 1995; Cox, 1999a). Patients will describe their pre-morbid lifestyle as being characterized by perfectionism, and high standards for work performance, responsibility and personal conduct, often placing great value on the opinion of others (Surawy et al., 1995).

Prior to the onset of CFS a person usually experiences a combination of psychosocial stress and an acute 'flu-like' illness (Sharpe et al., 1997; Kormaroff and Buchwald, 1998). The main precipitators or triggers that have been identified are a combination of:

- viral infections;
- significant internal and external stressors;
- overwork.

(Surawy et al., 1995)

The significant stressors will be those that place severe demands on the person or lead to depletion of their personal resources or both. A minor illness may then act as the final precipitating event or as a 'last straw' that tips the person into ill health (Surawy et al., 1995; Cox and Findley, 1998). For most patients it appears to be a combination of factors.

In the same way as the illness will have been triggered by certain factors there will be perpetuators of the illness. These are often similar to the precipitators, usually stress and recurrent infections, and the patterns that can develop in response to the symptoms (Joyce and Wessely, 1996; Cox, 1999a).

Therefore, once a state of fatigue is established, cognitive, behavioural, emotional, physiological and social factors may act to perpetuate it, such as:

* unhelpful beliefs;
* ineffective coping behaviour;
* negative mood states;
* social problems;
* pathophysiological processes.

(Surawy et al., 1995; Sharpe et al., 1996)

A vicious cycle then ensues, which traps the patients in chronic illness.

Inconsistent activity, and illness beliefs and fears about symptoms can fuel the illness (Joyce and Wessely, 1996; Sharpe et al., 1997). A person with CFS will not recover if he/she only has prolonged rest or pushes him/herself to the absolute limit (Joyce and Wessely, 1996). Rest can bring about short-term relief but in the longer term reduces activity tolerance (Cox and Findley, 1994). Conversely, strenuous activity following prolonged periods of rest has been shown to increase symptoms that perpetuate and reinforce activity avoidance behaviour (Butler et al., 1991). From this fluctuation between bursts of activity and prolonged rest, the pattern of activity has been described as the 'see-saw' effect, or peaks and troughs (Joyce and Wessely, 1996; Cox, 1999a).

The peaks of activity usually occur when patients with CFS feel well. They consequently tend to push themselves (peak) in an attempt to regain 'normal' function, and often go beyond their current fitness capacity so that they then have an excessive increase in symptomst. As a result of the increase in symptoms they take prolonged rest (trough) and so the cycle recurs (Sharpe et al., 1997; Cox, 1999a). This pattern happens on a daily and weekly basis, patients often carrying out most activity in the morning, then resting or sleeping each afternoon. Figure 1.3 describes this process diagrammatically.

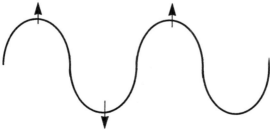

Not only occurs on a daily basis in response to symptoms but also weekly and monthly

Figure 1.3 The pattern of peaks and troughs of ability seen in CFS.

In addition, patients find that, owing to the fluctuations in symptoms, they may have two to three good days (peak) followed by two to three bad days (trough) (Cox, 1999a). Delayed fatigue and myalgia usually occur between 24 and 48 hours after any exertion in excess of the patient's current fitness level (Joyce and Wessely, 1996).

Following the observation of the impact on the CNS a cognitive model has been used when describing the precipitation and perpetuation of CFS (Surawy et al., 1995; Sharpe et al., 1996). Figure 1.4 shows the cycle as described by Surawy and colleagues (1995). In the absence of precise aetiology, using this model it is possible to see why cognitive approaches to the treatment of this illness have been used. The cognitive model constitutes a range of pragmatic approaches that effect change in an individual's ability and quality of life (Surawy et al., 1995; Sharpe et al., 1996; Deale et al., 1997).

Dysfunctional assumptions
If I am to be acceptable to myself and to others I must:
(a) achieve high standards of performance and responsibility
(b) be in control of my emotions and not display weakness

Pre-morbid behaviour
Strive for high standards. Do not complain or admit to any weakness. Neglect own needs

Critical incidents
Excessive demands (prolonged work stress) or reduced ability to meet demands (emotional consequences of life events, viral illness) leading to failure to meet requirements of assumptions.

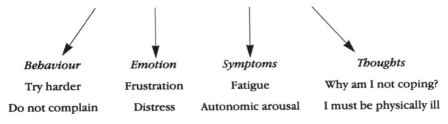

Behaviour	*Emotion*	*Symptoms*	*Thoughts*
Try harder	Frustration	Fatigue	Why am I not coping?
Do not complain	Distress	Autonomic arousal	I must be physically ill

Source: Surawy et al. (1995)

Figure 1.4 Theoretical cognitive model of aetiology and consequence of CFS.

It is from this model, combined with personal clinical experience and published evidence of effect, that the specific approach utilized by the author was developed, this is explained in detail in Section Four.

The following case vignette aims to illustrate a typical onset, presentation of the illness and consequent impact on an individual's life.

Case Vignette 1

Jane (aged 44) described the onset of her illness as starting five years prior to attendance. The onset followed a simple operation at her local hospital for removal of a tooth abscess. She stated that at the time she was under a lot of personal stress and had financial worries. Her mother had died in the previous year. On attendance at the occupational therapy session, she described her current symptoms as right-sided weakness and pain, sudden draining of energy, headache, generalized fatigue and a dry mouth. She was currently taking 50 mg of amitriptyline two hours prior to going to bed to assist with sleep disturbance. However, she said she still had difficulty getting off to sleep, woke frequently during the night and generally woke each morning feeling unrefreshed.

At the time of the onset of the illness she was working as a music therapist at her local centre for children with learning difficulties. She had stopped work two years ago as a result of the illness. Jane lived alone in her own house and could currently manage all her own personal care activities. However, she was reliant on her family and friends to complete domestic tasks, and was not currently able to socialize for longer than 10 minutes with one person in her own home. She was not able to maintain her normal social activities of attending the local church and visiting family and friends.

Prevalence and Prognosis

Prevalence

Overall, prevalence of CFS in the UK has been suggested to be 150 000 cases, with a 2:1 predominance of females compared with males (Wallace, 1991; Hinds and McCluskey, 1993). Table 1.1 shows the prevalence and prognosis from various studies of chronic fatigue around the world, and more specifically CFS. As can be seen from Table 1.1, more recent studies suggest a 3:1 predominance of females to males (Pawlikowska et al., 1994; Clark et al., 1995; Vercoulen et al., 1996) and the population prevalence of CFS to be between 0.3% and 1.5% (Bates et al., 1993; Pawlikowska et al., 1994; Buchwald et al., 1995; Wessely et al., 1995). In a sample taken from employees in an office building 0.9% met criteria for CFS (Shefer et al., 1997). Prevalence appears to be dependent on the case

Table 1.1 Prevalence and prognosis in studies of CF and CFS

Study	Setting and definition used	Duration of symptoms, age at outset and gender ratio (female: male)	Prevalence per 100 000 (type or definition)	Main outcome measures used	Assessment period	Conclusions
Bates et al., 1993	USA, primary care clinic, urban hospital-based general medicine practice n = 26 (CF) CFS n = 3 CDC Holmes et al., 1998 n = 4 UK, Sharpe et al., 1991 n = 10 Lloyd et al., 1990a	Duration > 6 months Mean age = 41.4 (CFS) Ratio 2:1	CDC = 0.3% UK = 0.4% Australia = 1.0% CFS only counts for small fraction of all cases of chronic, debilitating fatigue	Detailed history Physical examination Laboratory testing Psychiatric testing	1 year follow up	All 3 CFS patients remained fatigued Prevalence depends on case definition used
Buchwald et al., 1995	USA, health maintenance organization. n = 74 (CF) n = 3, CFS CDC Holmes et al., 1988	CFS = 6.1 years CF = 5.5 years Mean age = 41.3 (CFS) 44.9 (CF) Ratio 2:1	CFS = 75 to 267 (0.3%) CF = 1775 to 6321	SCL-90, SF-36, Brief fatigue inventory Symptom questionnaire Laboratory testing and physical examination	12 months 24 months	All 3 CFS patients remained fatigued. CFS and CF had poorer functional status and greater psychological distress than controls

Study	Setting / sample	Demographics	Comments	Measure	Follow-up	Results
Clark et al., 1995	USA, tertiary care, chronic fatigue clinic, university medical school n = 78, 19 (24%) met CFS 1988 CDC criteria	CF = 5.5 years Mean age = 39.9 Ratio 3:1	None given	Self-report questionnaire	2½ years	32/78 (41%) rated moderate to complete recovery 7/19 (37%) CFS patients recovered Poor outcome associated with older age (>38), longer duration of symptoms (>1.5 years), multiple physical symptoms, lifelong dysthymia
David et al., 1990	UK, primary care 611 general practice attenders, 64 had fatigue of greater than 1 month, 1 had CFS	> 1 week to > 6 months Mean age men = 38.8 women = 33.2 Ratio 2.8:1	None given Fatigue common complaint among general practice attenders and can be severe	Fatigue questionnaire (Wessely, 1989)	Initial only	Prognosis: none given Patients attribute illness to physical, psychological and social stress
Gold et al., 1990	USA, virology clinic n = 26 with at least 9 months of fatigue with physical symptoms and raised EBV titres. n = 6 CFS, 1988 CDC	Duration of CF = 3.5 years Mean age = 34.4 Ratio 1.4:1	None given	Symptom score Patients' assessment of improvement	3 to 21 months, mean, 11.3 months	4/21 complete recovery 8/21 significantly improved CFS 3/5 improved Most patients improve over time

(contd)

Table 1.1 (contd)

Study	Setting and definition used	Duration of symptoms, age at outset and gender ratio (female: male)	Prevalence per 100 000 (type or definition)	Main outcome measures used	Assessment period	Conclusions
Hinds and McCluskey, 1993	Northern Ireland, immunology outpatient clinic $n = 393, 291$ returned	Mean duration 5.22 years Mean age = 33 Ratio 2:1 females to males	None given	Postal questionnaire	Unclear, up to 6 years follow up	54 (18.6%) fully recovered Younger patients and those with a shorter duration of symptoms more likely to recover
Kroenke, et al., 1988	USA, army primary care clinic CF $n = 102$	Mean duration = 3.3 years Mean age range 40–64 Ratio 1.4:1	24% in the clinic population	Symptom of fatigue (2 scales). Changes in medical condition, medications, number of visits and hospitalizations	1 year follow up	29 (28%) with CF improved Older age and greater disability, abnormal ESR and clinic visits associated with poorer outcome
Lloyd et al., 1990	Australia, community CFS $n = 42$ (CDC Holmes, 1988)	Mean duration = 30 months Mean age = 28.6 yrs Ratio 1.3:1, less in community than tertiary care	CFS = 37.1 cases	Interview Psychiatric and medical assessment	None	CFS affects young individuals from all social classes and causes considerable ill health and disability
McDonald, David et al., 1993	UK, primary care attenders	Duration = >1 year Mean age = 32.5	None given	Interview Physical history	1 to 5 months	Prognosis: none given

Study	Sample	Duration/Ratio	Criteria	Methods	Follow-up	Comments
	CF n = 77 of which CFS = 17 (Sharpe et al., 1991)	Ratio 3:1		and examination data Socio-demographic Fatigue questionnaire Attributions		Identification of persistent fatigue and management in primary care may prevent secondary disabilities seen in CFS
Pawlikowska et al., 1994	UK, 6 primary care practices in southern England CF n = 2798 of which 38 = CFS	Duration = 18% >6 months Mean age not given Ratio 3:1	None given Possible 1%	Fatigue questionnaire GHQ	Community survey	Prognosis: none given General fatigue continuous variable in community
Ridsdale et al., 1993	UK, general practice Fatigue n = 220 of which 59% possible CFS	Duration = > 3 months Mean age = 43 Ratio 1.3:1	None given	Clinical data Laboratory tests Fatigue questionnaire GHQ	2 weeks, 2 and 6 months	Poor prognosis duration of symptoms longer than 6 months and history of anxiety or depression
Sharpe et al., 1992	UK, infectious diseases clinic n = 144 unexplained fatigued (CFS)	Median duration = 25 months Median age = 34 Ratio 1.5:1	None given	Assessment and interview questionnaires on degrees of recovery and functional impairment	6 weeks to 4 years	Functional impairment associated with belief in a viral cause, avoiding alcohol, changing or leaving employment, belonging to a self-help organization and current emotional disorder 13 % fully recovered, 65% were functionally impaired

(contd)

Table 1.1 (contd)

Study	Setting and definition used	Duration of symptoms, age at outset and gender ratio (female: male)	Prevalence per 100 000 (type or definition)	Main outcome measures used	Assessment period	Conclusions
Vercoulen et al., 1996	Holland, hospital clinic CFS *n* = 246	Mean duration 8.4 years Mean age = 39 Ratio 3:1	None given	Subjective experience Psychological well-being Functional impairment (SIP) Sleep disturbances Avoidance behaviour Neuropsychological functioning Social interactions Sense of control and causal attributions	18 months	3% complete recovery, 17% reported improvement Predictors of improvement were subjective sense of control over symptoms, less fatigue, shorter duration of complaints and a relative absence of physical attributions
Wessely et al., 1995	UK, primary care CF *n* = 100 CFS *n* = 12 (CDC, 1994)	Mean duration = 6 months Mean age = 32.7 Ratio 2:1	1.5 % Onset linked to previous fatigue and psychological disorder	Fatigue questionnaire GHQ CFS checklist Psychological assessment MOS short form	6 months' follow up	No evidence to suggest that common viral infections are associated with CFS in primary care

| Wilson et al., 1994a | Australia, university hospital referral centre CFS *n* = 103 (CDC, 1988) | Mean duration = 9.2 years Mean age = 42.2 Ratio 2.5:1 | None given | Somatic symptoms Structured interview Functional questionnaire Karnofsky performance index | Follow up mean 3.2 years after initial assessment | 6% complete recovery, 63% improved Psychological factors such as illness attitudes and coping are predictors of long-term outcome Strong conviction in a physical disease associated with poor outcome |

CFS = chronic fatigue syndrome
CF = chronic fatigue
CDC = Centre for Disease Control.

definition used. With three different CFS definitions (Holmes et al., 1988; Lloyd et al., 1990a; Sharpe et al., 1991) the prevalence ranged from 0.3% to 1% (Bates et al., 1993). In a later study this figure was adjusted to 98 per 100 000 (Buchwald et al., 1995).

One of the problems with many of the studies carried out on prevalence to date is possible selection bias. Almost all are based on tertiary care samples of patients, with patients often making their own diagnosis prior to seeking help (Wessley, 1995a). The more recent UK study in primary care (Pawlikowska et al., 1994) would appear to give the most realistic prevalence figure to date of 1%; however, in the same study only 0.2% thought that they had CFS (ME). Wessely (1995a) has stated that the 'systematic surveys that are now being published are beginning to suggest that CFS represents a substantial but neglected public health problem' (p. 142).

In the general population, chronic fatigue is a common complaint in primary care practice attendees with 18–27% (Kroenke et al., 1988; David et al., 1990; Bates et al., 1993; Pawlikowska et al., 1994) complaining of fatigue. However, only one in 10 of those patients would fulfil the criteria for CFS (Wessely et al., 1995).

The studies that have been completed in primary care do not indicate the higher predominance of professionals often seen in specialist secondary and tertiary referral centres and indicate no effect of sex or social class (Lloyd et al., 1990a; Wessely et al., 1995). The ratio of females to males in primary care also appears to be less than in secondary and tertiary care, with a ratio of 2:1 rather than 3:1 (Lloyd et al., 1990a). Lloyd and colleagues (1990a) conclude that the disorder is relatively common, affecting young adults in an approximately equal sex distribution. The most common time to develop the syndrome is in the peak productive years, with resulting disability persisting for prolonged periods of time.

Differences have been noted between the populations seen in primary and tertiary care (Euba et al., 1996). In particular, women are over represented in hospital samples. Gender could therefore be a weak risk factor for CFS. Overall, men have a worse perception of their health. Hospital cases often report less psychological distress (Euba et al., 1996), despite having more severe levels of fatigue. Self-diagnosis is more common in tertiary centres and a substantial number of patients are referred to specialists who do not fulfil the criteria for CFS (Wilson et al., 1994a). All these differences would need to be taken into consideration when evaluating a hospital CFS population.

Prognosis

Evidence of effective treatments for CFS is limited (Sharpe et al., 1996; Deale et al., 1997; Fulcher and White, 1997) and overall prognosis and recovery rate have been reported as generally extremely poor (Wessely, 1995a).

In 1988, Behan and Behan described the outcome of patients referred to a neurology service as follows:

> Most cases do not improve, give up their work and became permanent invalids, incapacitated by excessive fatigue and myalgia. (p.164)

There is evidence to support such gloomy outcomes. As can be seen from Table 1.1, studies over varying time scales of six months' to three years' follow up have indicated that with no intervention or management only 3–37% were fully recovered (Kroenke et al., 1988; Sharpe et al., 1992; Hinds and McCluskey, 1993; Wessely, 1995a; Vercoulen et al., 1996). However, with active medical care in a specialist CFS clinic 63% of patients were improved at a mean of 3.2 years' follow up, although only 6% had recovered completely (Wilson et al., 1994a). Those with chronic fatigue alone rather than CFS appear to show greater improvement, with 25% reporting resolution of their fatigue at one-year follow up (Buchwald et al., 1995). This may have an implication for the research design used to examine treatment methods and may indicate the fluctuating nature of the illness. Assessment may need to be carried out on a number of occasions to gain a true picture of improvement and recovery rather than just one or two time slots (Ray et al., 1997).

Patients with a subjective sense of control over symptoms, less fatigue, shorter duration of symptoms and an absence of physical attributions are more likely to improve (Sharpe et al., 1992; Vercoulen et al., 1996). In specialist settings poor prognosis appears to be associated with older age (Kroenke et al., 1988), the strength of physical attribution (Wilson et al., 1994a) and current emotional disorder (Euba et al., 1996). Psychological factors such as illness attitudes and coping appear to be predictors of long-term outcome (Wilson et al., 1994a; Vercoulen et al., 1996), in that belief in a physical cause, behavioural disengagement and coping mechanisms may effect recovery. Beliefs about illness could be considered important predictors of behaviour and desire to participate in rehabilitation (Joyce et al., 1997). Longitudinal studies that examine psychobiological relations between psychological distress and coping style, immunological function and the natural course of CFS are needed (Wilson et al., 1994a).

Chapter 2
The History of Chronic Fatigue Syndrome

When reviewing the history of chronic fatigue, for a similar group of symptoms to those seen today in chronic fatigue syndrome (CFS), there appear to have been a significant number of different titles used over the years (Acheson, 1959; Henderson and Shelokov, 1959; Parish, 1978; Behan and Behan, 1988; Wessely, 1990, 1991; Gilliam, 1992; Thomas, 1993).

These are:

1869 = neurasthenia;
1894 = fibrositis;
1906 = neurasthenia/ mild melancholia;
1934 = acute anterior poliomyelitis;
1937 = abortive poliomyelitis;
1948 = Iceland disease/Akureyri disease;
1950 = epidemic neuromyasthenia;
1952 = neuritis vegetativa epidemica;
1955 = encephalomyelitis/Royal Free disease;
1956 = benign myalgic encephalomyelitis;
1960 = chronic Epstein–Barr infection;
1978 = myalgic encephalomyelitis;
1984 = post-viral fatigue syndrome; Coxsackie B virus infection; Lake Tahoe disease;
1986 = 'yuppie flu';
1988 = chronic fatigue syndrome (USA: chronic fatigue and immune deficiency syndrome);
1996 = chronic fatigue syndrome (worldwide).

In the 20th century, there also appear to have been a number of epidemic outbreaks associated with similar symptoms, as opposed to the sporadic form seen today. Table 1.2 reports the epidemics reported over the years (Acheson, 1959; Henderson and Shelokov, 1959; Parish, 1978; Wessely, 1990, 1991; Wessely and Thomas, 1990; Gilliam, 1992; Hyde, 1992b; Thomas, 1993).

Table 2.1 Epidemic outbreaks

Year	Location studied	Reported cases	Nature of outbreak
1934	USA: Los Angeles, California	198	Hospital staff and community
1936	USA: Fond-du-Lac, Wisconsin	35	Convent candidates and novices
1937	Switzerland: Erstfeld	130	Soldiers
	Switzerland: Frohburg	28	Patients and staff
1939	England: Harefield	7	Hospital staff
	Switzerland: Degersheim	73	Soldiers
1945	USA: Pennsylvania	?	University hospital
1948–49	Iceland (Akureyri Disease)	1090	Community
1949–51	S. Australia: Adelaide	800	Community
1950	USA: Louisville, Kentucky	37	Student nurses
	USA: Upper New York State	19	Community
1952	England: Middlesex Hospital	14	Student nurses
	Denmark: Copenhagen	70+	Community
	USA: Lakeland, Florida	27	Community
1953	England: Coventry	13	Hospital staff and community
	USA: Rockville, Maryland	50	Student nurses and community
1954	USA:Tallahassee, Florida	450	Community
	USA: Seward, Alaska	175	Community
	Germany: Berlin	7	Barracks group
1954–55	S. Africa: Johannesburg	14	Community
1955	England: Dalston, Cumbria	?	Community
	England: Royal Free Hospital	300	Hospital staff
	W. Australia: Perth	?	Community
	Wales: Gilfach Goch	?	Community
	England: East Ham, London	?	Community
	S. Africa: Durban	140	Hospital staff and community
1955–56	Sierra Leone: Segbwema	?	Community
1956	USA: Ridgefield, Connecticut	70	Community
	USA: Punta Gorda, Florida	124	Community
	USA: Pittsfield, Massachusetts	7	Community
1956–57	Engand: Coventry	7	Community
1958	Greece: Athens	27	Student nurses
1959	England: Newcastle-upon-Tyne	?	Community
1961–62	USA: New York State	?	Convent
1964–65	USA: Galveston County	?	Community
1969	USA: New York State	?	University medical centre

Table 2.1 (contd)

Year	Location studied	Reported cases	Nature of outbreak
1970–71	England: Great Ormond Street Hospital, London	?	Hospital staff
1975	USA: Sacramento, California	200	Hospital staff
1976	Ireland: South West	?	Community
1979	England: Southampton	10	Community
1980–81	Scotland: Ayrshire	?	Rural practice
1980–83	Scotland: Helensburgh	?	GP practice
1983–84	New Zealand: West Otago	28+	Community
1984	USA: Lake Tahoe, Nevada	?	Teachers and pupils
1985	USA: Lyndonville, New York	?	Community

To review the history of CFS the information has been grouped into blocks of years: pre-1934, 1934–54, 1955–77, 1978–87, 1988–93 and 1994 to date.

Pre-1934

Looking back in history (*c.* 16th century) there is some reference to an illness like CFS, such as 'The English Sweats' (Henry VIII). Anne Boleyn is cited as being a sufferer. In 1854, from the age 35 to 60 years, Florence Nightingale is reported as suffering from:

* chest pain;
* headaches;
* rapid muscle fatigue;
* persistent upper back pain;
* being unable to concentrate if more than one person was present in the room.

(Hyde, 1992a)

In the American Civil War there was an illness termed 'Soldiers' Disease' for which the treatment was bedrest and hypernutrition for several months (Wessely, 1991; Hyde, 1992a). Prior to 1934 the syndrome was specified as having fatigue as its core symptom, and was described as being brought on by mere thought of exertion or by the anticipation of any task. The signs were cited as worry, fatigue and exhaustion (Wessely, 1990). It was commoner in educated and professional classes. In 1880, Beard listed over 70 symptoms with special attention being paid to specific areas:

* cardiac;
* gastrointestinal;

- temperature regulation;
- paraesthesiae;
- pain syndromes.

(Wessely, 1991)

The term 'neurasthenia' arrived between 1860 and 1880 and was referred to as the 'disease of the century' (Wessely, 1990, 1991). It was thought to derive from central exhaustion due to overwork, toxins, or metabolic or infective insults. In the early years the illness created a neurological paradigm. In the 1900s it was viewed as a psychological rather than a physical illness, and in due course was replaced by new psychiatric diagnoses of anxiety and depression (Wessely, 1990, 1991). Neurasthenia was described as the individual being the subject of fatigue or irritability beyond the reasonable results of mental or physical exertion and thereby partially or wholly incapacitated for his [sic] ordinary occupation or from the enjoyment of life (Hall, 1905).

Prior to 1906, it was viewed only as a disease of the upper classes. By 1906 it was viewed mainly as a disease of the lower social classes. Diagnosis was made 'for the comfort of the relatives and peace of mind of the patient' (Wessely, 1991, p. 925).

'Organicists' such as Beard argued that affective changes were an understandable reaction to the illness (Wessely, 1991). Weir Mitchell, an American founder of neurology, reaffirmed this, stating that it was impossible that neurasthenia could be:

...malady of the mind alone...as depression could not be an explanation for his condition, since he had no depression that was abnormal or unreasonable.
(Wessely, 1991, p. 922)

The 'rest cure' was first advocated by Weir Mitchell as the treatment of choice and remained popular for about 30 years (Wessely, 1991; Sabin and Dawson, 1993). By 1914 the observation that neurasthenia frequently followed an infection (influenza) was widely acknowledged (Wessely, 1991). By 1926 there had been a move from neuroses to psychoneuroses. By the 1930s physicians generally used descriptive labels, such as chronic nervous exhaustion, tired, weak, toxic, the main emphasis still being on psychological mechanisms (Wessely, 1990, 1991).

1934–54

In 1934 an epidemic was recorded in Los Angeles County Hospital (Gilliam, 1992; see Table 2.1) whereby all doctors and nurses were affected. In an attempt to treat their symptoms they were injected with immune prophylactic globulin. Their symptoms were described as:

- relapsing muscle weakness;
- inability to work;
- unusual pain syndromes;
- personality changes;
- memory loss;
- hysterical episodes;
- vertigo;
- major temperature fluctuations;
- pain in limbs;
- nausea;
- aphasia.

It was entitled *atypical poliomyelitis*, as the infective trigger was thought to be poliomyelitis. There appeared to be two forms of onset: acute and gradual. A greater predominance was noted in females. The 'sufferers' were often later labelled as 'malingerers' or as having 'compensationitis'. In 1968 Marinacci, when discussing the events of 1934, stated: 'this attitude often produced a conflict between the patient and the attending medical staff, and the patients were transferred from clinic to clinic and from department to department' (Hyde, 1992b, p. 127). Fourteen to 18 years later 21 of those originally affected were examined. Their main complaints were recurring:

- fatigue;
- pain;
- some muscle spasms (cervical and lumbrosacral);
- persistence of symptoms;
- impaired memory.

Many were paralysed and in wheelchairs (Hyde, 1992b).

1955–77

In 1955, at the Royal Free Hospital in London (Compston, 1978; see Table 2.1), 200 cases of an unknown illness were identified with the following range of symptoms:

- headache;
- sore throat;
- malaise;
- lymphadenopathy;
- lassitude;
- vertigo;

- pain in limbs;
- nausea;
- dizziness;
- stiff neck;
- pain in back/chest;
- depression;
- abdominal pain;
- vomiting;
- diplopia;
- tinnitus;
- diarrhoea.

The duration of hospital inpatient treatment varied from less than one month ($n = 114$) to greater than three months ($n = 14$). Two years following the episode only four patients still had marked physical disability.

When comparing the 1934 and 1955 outbreaks, Parish (1978) found that the triggers in both appeared to be a virus. Both appeared to be a systemic illness, distinguished in many patients by a prolonged convalescence, and portrayed by mental changes, particularly depression, autonomic disturbances, a profound tendency to fatigue easily and relapses of the original features of the illness.

In 1959, Donald Acheson described the symptoms of the illness as headache, low or absent fever, myalgia, paresis with symptoms or signs suggestive of damage to the brain; in essence, mental symptoms. He also noticed a higher frequency in women, a predominantly normal cerebrospinal fluid, and that sufferers were prone to relapses. There were a number of titles now being given to the illness such as benign myalgic encephalomyelitis, Iceland (Akureyri) disease and epidemic neuromyasthenia. It was observed to be a frequent occurrence among young female nurses in hospital epidemics while patients remained unaffected, which writers at the time found surprising (Acheson, 1959). Acheson (1959) made the following observations. The common symptoms were:

- generalized severe headache;
- stiffness in neck and back;
- pain in muscles of neck, shoulders and limbs that varied in intensity and was aggravated by exertion.

The pain was often agonizing and unresponsive to opiates. When the pain was severe it was accompanied by exquisite muscle tenderness, tender nerve trunks and skin sensitivity. He also noted muscular twitching, cramps, low fever and localized muscular weakness, which were variable in site and intensity. It was observed that full neurological examinations were rarely performed.

Many variations were seen between outbreaks. However, all were acute in duration with a range of four to 12 weeks. The acute symptoms often required hospitalization. Some people suffered relapses, although most recovered six months after onset. In some, relapses occurred with the menstrual cycle. Cyclical recurrences were seen in many of the epidemic patients $2^1/_2$ years after initial illness. The triggers appeared to be over-exertion and cold, damp weather (Acheson, 1959).

It was noted that in 39 patients with Iceland/Akureyri Disease (Sigurdsson and Gudmundsson, 1956) that six years after onset residual symptoms remained, although most had returned to work. Overall, there was a tendency towards slow improvement on a fluctuating course. The common symptoms remaining were nervousness, depression, fatigue, loss of memory, muscular pains, localized weakness and poor concentration. Headache and joint pain were also common, with occasional upper respiratory or gastrointestinal disturbances and paresis.

During this period, sporadic cases were also noted (Parish, 1978). The predominant symptoms described were:

- earache;
- headache;
- tinnitus;
- giddiness;
- muscular twitching;
- lassitude;
- cramps;
- low pyrexia;
- tremors;
- paresthesia;
- lymphadenopathy;
- muscle tenderness;
- stiffness of neck;
- paresis.

In the acute stage, people described terrifying dreams, panic states and hypersomnia. Later in the convalescent stage they described impairment of memory, difficulty in concentration and depression. Acheson (1959) drew the conclusion that this was a disorder of an infection spread by personal contact (Parish, 1978). There appeared to be a predominance in the medical and nursing professions, often with complete recovery within three months. The Royal Free epidemic was thought to be a manifestation of mass hysteria (Compston, 1978, discussing McEvedy and Beard, 1970).

By 1960, US reports linked chronic fatigue with the Epstein–Barr virus (EBV) (Wessely, 1991). There was thought to be central nervous system (CNS) involvement because of the common cognitive symptoms of diplopia, paraesthesia, unsteadiness, vertigo, blurring of vision, emotional lability, impairment of memory and concentration, terrifying nightmares and over-elaborated recital of symptoms.

1978–87

In 1978, Ramsey noted three types of response to the condition: complete recovery; recovery but prone to relapses; no recovery at all.

In 1991, Wessely noted that from 1978 to 1988 there was a shift from epidemic to sporadic cases, and an apparent change in the character of the illness. Persistent severe fatigue increased in importance in the sporadic cases, to become the hallmark of the disease. Contagion disappeared, but the prognosis worsened. In the 1980s the ME Association became Britain's fastest growing charity. In 1986 Professor Edwards and colleagues in Manchester, England separated peripheral fatigue from central fatigue, indicating that this central fatigue was manifested by deficits in the organization, integration and motivation of muscle action rather than dysfunction beyond the neuromuscular junction (Wessely, 1990). This finding added to the growing body of knowledge that the illness dysfunction lay within the CNS.

1988–93

From 1988 to 1993 depression was associated as a secondary phenomenon, distinguishable from clinical depression, as patients with CFS were less likely to report feelings of guilt, unworthiness and self-blame (Thomas, 1993). Subjective central fatigue was noted. Thomas stated that the illness appears to:

> ...reflect a complex interaction between cerebral dysfunction, trigger factors, and social attitudes and is complicated by secondary symptoms. (Thomas, 1993, p. 1558)

By 1988 the term chronic fatigue syndrome was introduced in the USA and Australia (Wessely, 1991). The triggers of overload due to viruses, pollution, stress and immune dysfunction were being suggested. In the USA the main viral trigger appeared to be EBV; in the UK it was cited as the enteroviruses such as poliovirus and Coxsackie (Dowsett et al., 1990).

From 1990 attention switched from muscle to brain (CNS). Wessely (1991) noted that the wheel had turned from peripheral, via central, to psychological explanations. He stated that patients felt that doctors did not take them seriously, i.e. it was all in the mind. The hysteria theory provoked anger and was often refuted (cf. 1955 epidemic description by McEvedy and Beard, 1970). Wessely (1990) warned of a need to ensure the syndrome was separated from other known conditions such as abnormal illness behaviour. Wessely and Thomas (1990) stated that:

> It cannot be overemphasised that the problem of epidemics has little or no relation to the problem posed by isolated cases in the community. Evidence of a psychological origin for epidemics neither proves nor disproves the aetiology of sporadic cases. (p. 115)

1994 to date

In the last few years much attention has been paid to the specific diagnostic criteria (Fukuda et al., 1994) as cited in Figure 1.2. In 1996, following the publication of the Report of the Royal Colleges of Psychiatrists, Physicians and General Practitioners (1996) on CFS, the name chronic fatigue syndrome was accepted in the UK as the diagnostic title. The Royal Colleges' report (1996) recommended ceasing to use the term myalgic encephalomyelitis or ME as it had not been operationally defined and could mislead patients into believing they have a serious and specific pathological process affecting muscles and brain (p.6).

In a 10-year follow-up study of 21 of the original 28 patients reported in the West Otago outbreak (1983–84) in New Zealand (see Table 2.1) it was found that a high proportion of patients had recovered (Levine et al., 1997). This therefore suggested that epidemic CFS has a better prognosis than sporadic cases.

In conclusion, CFS is not new. What was once described as neuraesthenia appears to be the modern-day CFS. Having considered the history of what we now know as CFS there does appear to have been a change in the clinical nature of the syndrome over time. The evidence suggests that dysfunction lies within the CNS (see Chapter 1), and though epidemics are still occasionally reported most cases now appear to be sporadic with a poor prognosis (Wessely, 1991).

Section Two will discuss and consider the assessment process and pharmacological treatment available in the management of CFS.

Section Two:
The Clinical Management of Chronic Fatigue Syndrome

The management of chronic fatigue syndrome (CFS) involves accurate definition and assessment to ensure appropriate diagnosis and that consequent treatment is tailored to the individual concerned (Wilson et al., 1994b; Sharpe et al., 1997). The following two chapters aim to consider the current clinical assessment process and treatment available in the pharmacological management of CFS.

Chapter 3
The Clinical Assessment of Chronic Fatigue Syndrome

Owing to the lack of any consistent abnormalities being identified, laboratory tests have been shown to be generally unhelpful in the diagnostic process of chronic fatigue syndrome (CFS) (Valdini et al., 1989; Lane et al., 1990). Therefore a clinical evaluation process emphasizing exclusion of alternative conditions is paramount, as failure to identify an underlying illness that could cause fatigue could influence the success of treatment (Fukuda et al., 1994; Hickie, Lloyd and Wakefield, 1995). However, laboratory tests that assist in the exclusion of other aetiological possibilities and/or concurrent non-causative pathology including treatable co-morbidity consequently need to form part of the evaluation process (Fukuda et al., 1994; Hickie et al., 1995).

Laboratory Tests

A minimum battery of tests to assist in the assessment process has been suggested as:

- complete blood cell count with manually performed differential white blood cell count;
- erythrocyte sedimentation rate;
- blood chemistry;
- thyroid stimulating hormone (supersensitive assay);
- antinuclear antibodies;
- circulating immune complexes;
- immunoglobulin levels (IgG, IgA and IgM).

These tests are thought to be helpful to support the diagnosis and rule out any other diseases that could produce chronic fatigue (Buchwald and Kormaroff, 1991; Fukuda et al., 1994). Additional tests may be indicated by the clinical history or examination on an individual basis to confirm or exclude another diagnosis, such as multiple sclerosis or sleep apnoea (Fukuda et al., 1994; Hickie, Lloyd and Wakefield, 1995).

The Multi-dimensional Assessment Approach

In the absence of specific tests for CFS, a multi-dimensional approach to its assessment has been suggested that includes subjective assessment of behavioural, emotional, social and cognitive aspects such as:

- fatigue;
- mood disturbance;
- functional status;
- sleep disorder;
- global well-being;
- pain (Schluederberg et al., 1992; Vercoulen et al., 1994).

However, the use of multiple measures increases the complexity of the assessment and because of the length of most instruments they are likely to remain as research tools primarily. They tend not to be used routinely by clinicians owing to the difficulty of use in clinical practice (Buchwald et al., 1997). The use of measures is discussed further in Chapter 10.

High rates of concurrent psychiatric disorder have been noted in a primary care study (Wessely et al., 1996). The General Health Questionnaire (GHQ) has been suggested as a useful screening tool for psychiatric disorder in CFS as it is short and easy to administer (Buchwald et al., 1997). Johnson and colleagues (1996) emphasize the importance of screening for concurrent psychiatric disorder as they found that by thorough assessment, patients with CFS and concurrent depressive illness could be differentiated from those without depression, therefore enabling appropriate treatment. Additionally, in a previous study, two-thirds of patients reporting to a fatigue clinic appeared to have psychiatric disorders as the cause of their chronic fatigue (Manu et al., 1988). These studies highlight the importance of the need for both physical and mental health examinations as suggested in Figure 3.1 (Fukuda et al., 1994; Hickie et al., 1995).

The Assessment of Persistent Fatigue

Figure 3.1 indicates a simple approach to the assessment of persistent fatigue as described by Hickie et al. (1995) and defined by the International CFS study group (Fukuda et al., 1994). The most important aspect of the assessment process is a carefully taken history including:

History
- Record the medical and psychosocial circumstances at onset of symptoms
- Assess previous physical and psychological health
- Elucidate any underlying medical disorder (e.g. fevers, weight loss, dyspnoea)
- Record the duration of symptoms
- Assess the impact of the symptoms on the patient's lifestyle

Characteristic symptoms of CFS include: fatigue, myalgia, arthralgia, impaired memory and concentration

Physical examination
- Seek abnormalities to suggest an underlying medical disorder
  - hypothyroidism
  - chronic hepatitis
  - chronic anaemia
  - neuromuscular disease
  - sleep apnoea syndrome
  - occult malignancy, etc.

The physical examination in patients with CFS characteristically shows no abnormalities

Mental state examination
- Past or family history of psychiatric disorder, notably depression or anxiety
- Past history of frequent episodes of medically unexplained symptoms
- Past history of alcohol or substance abuse
- Current symptoms: depression, anxiety, self-destructive thoughts, and use of over-the-counter medications
- Assess for current signs of psychomotor retardation
- Evaluate psychosocial system

CFS patients have depressive symptoms but not guilt, suicidal ideation or observable psychomotor slowing

Laboratory investigation
- Screening tests:
  - urinalysis
  - blood count and differential
  - erythrocyte sedimentation rate
  - renal function tests

  liver function tests
  calcium, phosphate
  random blood glucose
  thyroid function tests
- Additional investigations as clinically indicated

The diagnosis of CFS is primarily one of exclusion of alternative conditions

Chronic fatigue syndrome
- *Unexplained, persistent or relapsing chronic fatigue lasting six or more consecutive months (see full definition in Chapter 1 Figure, 1.2)*
- *Four or more of the symptoms listed in the definition*

Source: Adapted from Hickie et al. (1995)

Figure 3.1 Approach to the assessment of persistent fatigue.

- the patient's presenting complaints;
- history of the illness;
- current situation;
- family and personal history;
- past medical history;
- pre-morbid personality and lifestyle (Sharpe et al., 1997; Fuller and Morrison, 1998).

In particular, it is necessary to record:

- the preceding events and circumstances at the onset of symptoms, such as stress or illness;
- the complete list of symptoms;
- duration of the illness;
- previous physical and psychological health;
- the impact of the symptoms on the patient's lifestyle;
- their understanding of the illness (Hickie et al., 1995; Clements et al., 1997).

Patients with CFS have been noted to generally report more life events in the year prior to the onset of the illness (Salit, 1997). It is extremely important to discuss the patient's understanding of his/her illness in order to gain an impression of the strength in which the patient holds his/her illness beliefs, as this could have an impact on the outcome of any future treatment (Sharpe et al., 1997). Patients who hold a purely physical attribution for their symptoms have consistently been shown to have a poor outcome (Sharpe et al., 1992; Vercoulen et al., 1996).

The list of the symptoms as cited within the definition criteria (see Chapter 1, Figure 1.2) has been shown to be useful to check as the patient gives a history (Fukuda et al., 1994; Fuller and Morrison, 1998). By doing so the list may reveal the presence of symptoms related to other disorders such as major depression (Sharpe et al., 1997).

Leitch (1994) points out, though, that history taking takes time and patience. However, if employed to the full it enables the establishment of a doctor–patient relationship which may in itself be therapeutic (Leitch, 1994; Clements et al., 1997). Sharpe and colleagues (1997) emphasize this point by discussing the importance of forming a positive relationship with the patient, in order to form a basis for any future therapy. This is particularly important as patients may have had previous conflicting information about what is wrong with them, and need time for questions to be answered (Sharpe et al., 1997).

Chapter 4
The Pharmacological Management of Chronic Fatigue Syndrome

Antidepressants

Many pharmacological treatments have been proposed for chronic fatigue syndrome (CFS) over the years (Behan and Behan, 1988; Wessely, 1992; Leitch, 1994). Antidepressants are often cited as the treatment of choice (Joyce and Wessely, 1996). Many clinicians have found that low-dose tricyclic drugs (10–20 mg), particularly at bedtime, are beneficial in improving sleep and reducing the symptoms of CFS (Kormaroff and Buchwald, 1998). The justification for using antidepressants is based on the assumption that depression can be an understandable consequence of CFS. In addition, they act as broad-spectrum agents that can affect pain, sleep and energy (Sharpe et al., 1997). However, the few studies that have been completed do not give conclusive evidence of antidepressants' overall efficacy with CFS patients (Sharpe et al., 1997; Kormaroff and Buchwald, 1998).

Initial anecdotal evidence suggested that, for some patients with CFS, antidepressant therapy did assist in management and symptom reduction (Lynch et al., 1991). In particular:

- tricyclics such as amitriptyline or dothiepin;
- selective serotonin reuptake inhibitors (SSRIs) such as fluoxetine or paroxetine;
- monoamine oxidase inhibitors (MAOIs) such as moclobemide were suggested (Gantz and Holmes, 1989; Lynch et al., 1991).

Low-dose amitriptyline (25 mg) has been shown to be beneficial in the treatment of patients with fibromyalgia (Goldenberg et al., 1986) and has been cited frequently as improving sleep disturbance in patients with CFS (Gantz and Holmes, 1989; Goodnick and Sandoval, 1993; Kormaroff and Buchwald, 1998). However, although much has been written about the benefits of amitriptyline for CFS patients, no controlled trials have been completed to date (Kormoroff and Buchwald, 1998).

Some patients with CFS are unable to tolerate tricyclics even in low doses owing to sedation and anticholinergic effects such as dry mouth and blurred vision (Lynch et al., 1991; Wilson et al., 1994b). In general, patients with CFS are sensitive to the adverse effects of medication (Sharpe, 1991; Wilson et al., 1994b). Therefore, SSRIs such as fluoxetine (Prozac) have been used in the treatment of CFS as they have been noted to have fewer sedative and autonomic nervous system side-effects as compared wth the tricyclics (Lynch et al., 1991; Vercoulen et al., 1996). Clinical experience, especially in primary care, suggests that SSRIs appear to be better tolerated than tricyclic antidepressants (Martin et al., 1997).

Research on cerebral serotonergic abnormality in patients with CFS provides a specific argument to support the use of SSRIs in CFS (Demitrack et al., 1991; Cleare et al., 1995; Chapter 1, 'Aetiology: Central Nervous System'). Behan and colleagues (1994) in an open uncontrolled study of the SSRI sertraline administered for six months at a dose of 50 mg per day, reported that it was well tolerated and most patients improved in terms of fatigue, muscle pain, sleep disturbance and depression (although none had major depression). However, in one randomized controlled trial (RCT) of fluoxetine compared with placebo completed in CFS (Vercoulen et al., 1996), after eight weeks' treatment of 20 mg daily dose, fluoxetine did not have a beneficial effect on any characteristic of CFS. Interestingly, in an RCT of fluoxetine at the same dose, graded exercise and placebo, fluoxetine was more effective in reducing Hospital Anxiety and Depression (HAD) scale scores (Zigmond and Snaith, 1983) than placebo at three months but not at six months (Wearden et al., 1998). The study by Wearden and colleagues (1998) perhaps provides modest support for the use of fluoxetine in CFS with depression, and the evidence suggests treatment effect with SSRIs may take longer than eight weeks (Behan et al., 1994; Wearden et al., 1998).

It has been postulated that CFS is a disorder of reduced central sympathetic drive, and that low-dose treatment with a MAOI such as phenelzine (Nardil) may be beneficial (Natelson et al., 1996). The use of MAOIs in the treatment of CFS is further supported by their specificity in treating atypical depression (Liebowitz et al., 1988). Natelson and colleagues (1996) administered a maximum dose of phenelzine that was only 25% of the therapeutic dose for depression, and therefore reasoned that it would not have an anti-depressant effect. The drug was administered to CFS patients without depression over a four-week period with a two-week placebo run-in. Although more treated patients noted improvement on more tests than the majority of placebo control patients, the improvement was not striking (Natelson et al., 1996). The length of time experienced by clinicians to show an effect appears to vary (Wessely et al., 1998; Kormoroff and Buchwald, 1998), thus four weeks may have been an insufficient period.

Early clinical evidence suggested that moclobemide (a reversible MAOI) had a moderate or marked response in a small number of patients (Wilson et al., 1994b). In an open study of the effects of moclobemide in patients with CFS, the results indicated that it may be useful for patients with a co-morbid major depressive disorder, as 50% of these patients rated themselves as better compared with 19% who were not depressed (White and Cleary, 1997). However, White and Cleary (1997) noted that eight weeks rather than six weeks of treatment and starting at a higher dose may have enhanced efficacy in patients without co-morbid depression.

It has been suggested as there is insufficient evidence to support the use of antidepressants as a first-line treatment of CFS, and that their use should be restricted to situations where there is either: clear-cut evidence of accompanying depression; and/or severe problems with muscle pain or sleep disturbance (Wessely et al., 1998). The choice of antidepressant is dependent on the effect required, such as sedation or change in mood (Wessely et al., 1998).

Other Treatments

Treatments other than antidepressants have been considered in CFS, although controlled trials are limited. As previously discussed (see Chapter 1, 'Aetiology: Immune Dysfunction') considerable attention has been given to the possible role of immune dysfunction in CFS (Wessely, 1995a). Lloyd and colleagues (1990b) reported that immunomodulatory treatment with three immunoglobulin infusions was effective in a significant number of patients with CFS (43%, 10/23) compared with placebo (12%, 3/26). They suggested that the results supporting the concept of an immunologic disturbance may be important in the pathogenesis of CFS (Lloyd et al., 1990b). However, in a later study of immunologic and psychologic therapy, patients with CFS did not demonstrate specific response to either treatment or a combination of treatment compared with placebo (Lloyd et al., 1993, see Table 5.1). Further study of intravenous immunoglobulin alone failed to replicate the findings of the previous study (Vollmer-Conna et al., 1997). It was concluded that intravenous immunoglobulin therapy cannot be recommended as a treatment for CFS (Vollmer-Conna et al., 1997).

Some patients with CFS have been shown to have slightly lower magnesium levels than healthy controls and treatment with magnesium may be beneficial, especially in respect of energy and emotional status (Cox et al., 1991). However, these results were much debated, with further studies failing to replicate the findings (Gantz, 1991; Deulofeu et al., 1991). It was suggested that clinicians should not use intramuscular magnesium sulphate unless a deficiency could be demonstrated in the patient (Gantz, 1991).

A study by Bou-Holaigah and colleagues (1995) supported the association of CFS with neurally mediated hypotension by reporting complete or near complete resolution of CFS symptoms after increasing dietary salt intake and taking fludrocortisone for one month. However, in a study carried out in an attempt to replicate the findings, Peterson and colleagues (1998) found that low-dose fludrocortisone did not provide conclusive evidence that it was of benefit to patients with CFS.

Conclusion

There is no definitive pharmacological management in the treatment of CFS to date. The tricyclic antidepressants, although still awaiting controlled trials, appear the most useful in controlling sleep disturbance, pain and mood (Sharpe et al., 1997; Wessely et al., 1998).

Section Three will discuss the current treatment approaches in CFS.

Section Three: Treatment Approaches in Chronic Fatigue Syndrome

Established treatment approaches specific to chronic fatigue syndrome (CFS) are limited (Sharpe et al., 1996; Cox, 1999a). The patient needs to be treated as an individual with his/her own specific triggers and perpetuators of CFS, i.e. the supposed causes and precipitators (Wessely, 1992; Chapter 1, 'Presentation') and pattern of daily activities identified (Cox and Findley, 1998; Cox, 1999a).

In general, the advice given to patients has been misleading (Wessely et al., 1989). Patients were often told to 'rest until symptoms subside' or to 'learn to live within their limits and modify their lifestyle' (Butler et al., 1991). All aspects of treatment need to be based on improving the patient's ability to manage his/her daily life and increase their overall functioning (Ho-Yen, 1990). The two main evidence-based treatment approaches that appear to warrant consideration are cognitive behavioural therapy and graded exercise.

Chapter 5
Cognitive Behavioural Therapy

Cognitive behavioural therapy (CBT) is a recent addition to psychological treatment. It appears to fill the gap between purely behavioural methods and dynamic psychotherapies, being directly concerned with 'faulty' thoughts and feelings (Enright, 1997).

The prognosis of those with chronic fatigue syndrome (CFS) has been cited to be poor (Kroenke et al., 1988; Hinds and McCluskey, 1993; Vercoulen et al., 1996; Chapter 1, 'Prognosis'). However, studies completed in the last five years have indicated that CBT intervention can change outcome in CFS patients (Sharpe et al., 1996; Deale et al., 1997; Table 5.1). The following section aims to outline the history and development of CBT and supports the reason for its use with CFS patients by means of a cognitive model. The empirical foundations of cognitive behavioural approaches can be traced back to the early part of the 20th century.

The Development of Behavioural and Cognitive Therapies

Work carried out in the late 19th and early 20th century identified two principles of animal learning and behaviour. The first was based on the work of Pavlov and other Russian physiologists. The phenomenon observed during their experiments become known as *classical conditioning*. The Russian investigators also found that emotional responses such as fear can be conditioned. The second principle, which derived from the observational work in the USA by Thordike, Tolman and Guthrie, became known as *operant conditioning* (Hawton et al., 1989). They identified the 'law of effect' following a series of experiments in which they found that if a particular behaviour was consistently followed by a reward the behaviour was more likely to occur again.

Skinner took the principle further by defining reinforcers. He described positive reinforcement as the situation where a behaviour occurs more frequently because it is followed by positive consequences, and negative reinforcement as the situation where the frequency of a behaviour increases because it is followed by omission of an anticipated aversive event. The term reinforcement therefore always refers to situations in which behaviour increases in frequency or strength. Decreases in frequency of a behaviour are associated with punishment and non-reward. When operant-conditioning principles are used in patient treatment, events are used as reinforcers that have previously being shown to change the behaviour in the desired direction (Hawton et al., 1989).

The 1960s saw an expansion in the application of behavioural treatments to a wide range of problems. The 1970s saw the full emergence of behaviour therapy, with numerous techniques being developed and experimentally validated. Behaviour therapy became the treatment of choice for many disorders, such as phobia, obsession and sexual dysfunction, with the use of operant and goal setting techniques in rehabilitation (Hawton et al., 1989). However, in the late 1960s and early 1970s dissatisfaction with the fixed methods of behavioural practice was encountered. In particular, Lazarus (1971) rejected what he believed to be mechanistic concepts underlying the practice of behaviour therapy (Hawton et al., 1989). This dissatisfaction resulted in attempts to add cognitive components to existing techniques, opening the way for the development and application of cognitive approaches. A major development in cognitive theory was the adoption in the 1970s of Lang's three-system approach of behavioural, cognitive/affective and physiological independent response systems. It was proposed that these systems, although linked, did not necessarily change at the same time (Hawton et al., 1989).

The first cognitive approach to create interest among behaviour researchers was 'self-instructional training' proposed by Meichenbaum in 1975. This approach had a simple theoretical basis. Meichenbaum suggested that behaviour change could be brought about by changing the instructions that patients gave themselves. The theory was that by changing the instructions, patients would move away from maladaptive and upsetting thoughts to more constructive healthy thoughts (Hawton et al., 1989). This was the basis of the more sophisticated cognitive therapy described by Beck (1976). Beck's cognitive therapy, which was similar to Ellis's (1962) rational emotive therapy, took time to become accepted but has now become the most important of the cognitive approaches (Hawton et al., 1989).

Beck (1976) proposed that the negative thinking so prominent in depression was not just a symptom but had a central role in the maintenance of depression. This implied that depression could be treated by helping patients to identify and modify their negative thoughts. Beck proposed that negative thinking originated in attitudes, or as he called them assumptions, which arose from experiences in early life (Enright, 1997). Assumptions could be positive and motivating but if held to extreme they could make the individual vulnerable to certain events and lead to the production of *'negative automatic thoughts'* (Beck, 1976; Hawton et al., 1989; Enright, 1997). The 'thoughts' related to concepts, opinions or ideas; 'automatic' meant they tended to appear suddenly of their own accord, without any conscious or deliberate effort; and 'negative' meant working against.

Such thoughts, Beck (1976) considered, lowered mood, which in turn increased the possible negative thoughts and produced a vicious circle. Once established, the negative thoughts could be very difficult to switch off and often appeared quite logical and plausible. However, Beck (1976) proposed that there were alternative ways of viewing things that would be more helpful and enable the person to feel better and do more.

In addition, Ellis (1962) introduced the concept of irrational beliefs, based on our own individual underlying beliefs and rules, which again if held to the extreme could influence behaviour. Beck (1976) extended the application of cognitive therapy to a wide range of emotional disorders. He identified a number of thinking styles, and these included cognitive deficiency, arbitrary inference, dichotomous thinking, magnification, over-generalization and personalization, all of which could have an influence on an individual's well-being (see Glossary for explanation of terms).

The Rationale for the Use of CBT with CFS

CBT is based on the theory that inaccurate unhelpful beliefs, ineffective coping behaviour, negative mood states, social problems and pathophysiological processes all interact to perpetuate illness (Sharpe et al., 1997). The cognitive model previously introduced (see Figure 1.4) indicates how these dysfunctional assumptions lead to the interaction of behaviour, emotion, symptoms and thoughts in CFS (Surawy et al., 1995). The positive effect of CBT has been shown in the treatment of other disorders such as:

- anxiety disorder;
- obsessional–compulsive disorder;
- panic disorder and agoraphobia;
- schizophrenia;
- depression;

- chronic pain (Andrews, 1996, see Table 5.1; Simons et al., 1986; Williams et al., 1993).

The expansion of CBT to many conditions other than depression was based on the premise that cognitive and behavioural factors are relevant to all human experience. Its application now ranges from depression to chronic pain (Williams et al., 1993; Enright, 1997).

Considerable attention is now being paid in psychiatry to thoughts and beliefs (cognitions) experienced in a wide variety of situations (Wessely, 1995c). CBT is based in the here and now, and the main goal of therapy is to help patients bring about desired changes in their lives. Cognitive (our conscious thoughts), attributional (belief about illness) and behavioural factors play a crucial role in determining outcome and mediating disability. Crucial to this argument is the basic assumption that what causes an illness is not always the same as what determines prognosis, hence treatment may not be determined by the nature of the initial insult (Wessely, 1995c; Chapter 1, 'Presentation').

Attribution is an individual's perception of fact, and can be viewed from a number of perspectives as shown in Figure 5.1. The aim of CBT is to make the attribution external and temporary rather than internal and permanent (Wessely, 1995c). At present the attribution of CFS is frequently associated with a belief that the condition is incurable, and that symptoms should be managed by rest (Wessely, 1995c; Clements et al., 1997). Attribution of illness can be formed through misinformation from the media, previous inappropriate advice from professionals and, with the increasing use of computers, the Internet.

	TEMPORARY	PERMANENT
INTERNAL		
EXTERNAL		

Source: Davies (1993)

Figure 5.1 Perspectives of attribution in cognitive therapy.

The 'rest cure' as a treatment for fatiguing illness has a long history (Wessely, 1991), and though it may have relieved symptoms in the short term, in the long term it created problems by reducing exercise tolerance and producing increased weakness, muscle wasting and cardiac and respiratory difficulties, together with increased sensitivity to activity (Greenleaf and Kozlowski, 1982; Sharpe and Wessely, 1998).

Physical illness attributions and the presence of an emotional disorder have been shown to be associated with disability in CFS at two-year follow up (Sharpe et al., 1992). This finding was replicated in the study by Wilson and colleagues (1994a) in that the belief in the illness being a physical disease was predictive of poor outcome. It has also been postulated that individual differences in beliefs and cognitions about CFS may influence the limits and boundaries CFS patients set in their level of functioning (Petrie et al., 1995). In particular, catastrophic thinking may be an important factor in determining disability within CFS (Petrie et al., 1995).

Over the last 10 years a cognitive theory of CFS has developed, in that certain factors and events are thought to precipitate, trigger and perpetuate the illness (Wessely et al., 1989; Surawy et al., 1995). This theory attempts to explain how certain life stresses may precipitate CFS in predisposed persons, and how cognitive, behavioural, physiological and social factors then interact to perpetuate the illness (Surawy et al., 1995, see Figure 1.4; Sharpe et al., 1997). In the presence of any long-term illness, it can be very difficult to retain a positive outlook in the face of prolonged disability, restriction of everyday life, and absence of a ready cure. The feelings associated with CFS, such as frustration, anger, irritability, anxiety, demoralization and profound change in mood, could therefore impair recovery (Surawy et al., 1995).

A study by Clements and colleagues (1997) found that most patients believed that they could control their symptoms to some degree but could not alter the course of the underlying disease process. The coping methods they described were resting, avoiding activity and reducing activity. Personal experience of feeling worse after activity was a major factor in the adoption of rest and avoidance (Ray et al., 1995; Clements et al., 1997). Therefore, interventions that either discourage avoidance of activity or enhance perceived control could benefit the course of the illness (Ray et al., 1997).

The cognitive behavioural model is therefore based on the understanding that thoughts, feelings and actions interlink with each other; what we do influences thoughts and feelings and, equally, the way we think can affect actions and feelings (Surawy et al., 1995). For example, thoughts such as 'I won't be able to do this properly' make it hard even to start anything. Equally, a person may find him/herself feeling worried, frustrated or helpless before or during an activity. These feelings are often linked to such thoughts, for example, as 'I can't imagine getting over this' or 'I might make myself worse', which are likely to contribute to feelings of fearfulness or helplessness that are not only distressing but could hold back that individual. Alternatively, thoughts such as 'I won't know whether I can get over this until I try' or 'I don't know whether I will feel worse, and I might even feel better' are likely to make a person feel optimistic and in control. In other words, a change in one area will often lead to a change in the others (Beck, 1976; Wessely, 1995c).

The cognitive model used to conceptualize the origin of CFS as suggested by Surawy and colleagues (1995), and illustrated in Figure 1.4, leads us to see that from the assumptions, a vicious cycle of alternating between effort and ineffectual rest is maintained by the attribution of symptoms to disease, and holds the patient in chronic illness.

The cornerstone of treatment is therefore the combination of CBT therapy with a cautious graded resumption of activity, using clearly defined, modest and predictable goals (Cox and Findley, 1994, 1998; Wessely, 1995c). Cognitive factors (beliefs about health and illness) and behavioural factors (the use of avoidance as a coping strategy) are important determining factors in the outcome of CFS. All contribute to the vicious cycle postulated by the group at King's College, London, UK (Wessely et al., 1989; Wessely, 1995c). In addition, because of the heterogeneous nature of CFS it is likely that a complex interaction of physiological, cognitive, behavioural and affective factors is responsible for its development and maintenance (Chalder et al., 1996; Chapter 1, 'Clinical Features and Presentation'). A cognitive behavioural model takes into account such factors and points towards effective treatment.

The pre-morbid personalities of patients with CFS are often characterized by:

- overactivity;
- overwork;
- achievement orientation;
- high standards for work performance (Surawy et al., 1995; Cox, 1999a).

Symptoms are perpetuated by physical illness attributions, unhelpful cognitions and schemes relating to perfectionism and coping strategies that involve avoiding or reducing activity (Chalder et al., 1996). CBT is used to modify these behaviours and the beliefs that may maintain disability and symptoms (Deale et al., 1997). The focus of CBT is therefore to break the link between the spiral of increasing fatigue, and reducing or stopping activity (Sharpe et al., 1996; Deale et al., 1997; Cox and Findley, 1998).

Table 5.1 shows the various ways in which CBT has been used in the management of CFS and indicates the conclusions and limitations of the studies. The randomized controlled trials that have been completed indicate that CBT leads to a reduction in functional impairment and improved fatigue in 70–73% of outpatients with CFS (Sharpe et al., 1996; Deale et al., 1997). Interestingly, the study by Lloyd and colleagues (1993) did not indicate significant improvement but was based on $3^1/_2$ to 6 hours of outpatient CBT compared with 13 to 16 hours in other studies (Sharpe et al., 1996; Deale et al., 1997). The non-randomized controlled studies completed indicated similar findings with 57–82% of inpatients and out-patients showing improvement at three months, six months and four years following intervention (Butler et al., 1991; Bonner et al., 1994; Cox and Findley, 1994; Chalder et al., 1996). These findings appear comparable to the response of patients with depression and chronic pain (Simons et al., 1986; Williams et al., 1993). However, as can be seen from Table 5.1 a variety of scales and comparison groups have been used in the studies cited, making comparison of the results difficult.

The Practice of CBT

CBT involves the achievement of mutually agreed activity targets. These are not prescriptive nor are they synonymous with graded exercises (Lloyd et al., 1993). Targets are chosen on the basis of avoidance. The targets could involve minimal activity and convey no ergonomic or physiological benefits. They may not be physical activities at all but may be designed to increase concentration (Chalder et al., 1995). The targets need to be consistent, predictable and achievable. In order to achieve these targets, rest must also be planned into the day and be consistent. The cognitive aspect is therefore to correct dysfunctional thinking and graded activity; the behavioural aspect is utilized to eliminate avoidance (Cox and Findley, 1994, 1998; Wessely, 1995c).

The details of the CBT programme are discussed with the patient before therapy begins, each session is planned, and therapy is usually time limited to achieve a specific outcome (Deale et al., 1997; Chapter 9). Symptoms, disability and risk factors are measured regularly throughout the therapy. CBT focuses on thinking, in particular maladaptive thinking styles, beliefs, rules and attributions. The approach is one of equal partnership between therapist and patient (Andrews, 1996; Sharpe et al., 1997). The approach is empirical, using clear goals, homework tasks and counselling skills.

At the start of therapy a thorough assessment is made and a history is taken, with consideration between the links of cognitive, behaviour, social

Table 5.1 CBT studies

Authors and title	Subject Nos	Type of study and length of follow up	Outcome measures	Results of trial	Conclusions	Limitations of the study
Deale et al. (1997) *Cognitive Behaviour Therapy for Chronic Fatigue Syndrome: A Randomized Controlled Trial* (UK)	60	RCT with final assessment at 6 months. 13 sessions of CBT or relaxation	General Health Survey – Short form, Work and Social Adjustment Scale, Long-term Goals Rating, Fatigue Problem Scale, Fatigue Questionnaire, General Health Questionnaire, Beck Depression Inventory, Global Self-ratings Scale, Assessor ratings, Illness attributions	19/27 improved in CBT group, 5/26 improved in relaxation group, 70% versus 19%	CBT was more effective than a relaxation control in the management of CFS. Improvements were sustained over 6 months of follow up	Use of a single therapist. Self-rated outcomes but no objectives measures exist for subjective symptoms
Chalder, Butler and Wessely (1996) *Inpatient Treatment of Chronic Fatigue Syndrome* (UK)	6	Before/after design — pre- and post-treatment and follow up. Therapy hours range 7–15 hr	Assessment, Targets, Social Adjustment Questionnaire, Fear Questionnaire, Beck Depression Inventory, Fatigue Scale	5 cases much improved, 4 of the 5 maintained improvement at 3 months, 2 were able to return to work	Unclear whether recovery due to therapist time, specific techniques or antidepressants. Unlikely to be due to chance	Not RCT, results therefore should be interpreted with caution

Study	N	Method	Measures	Results	Comments
Sharpe et al. (1996) *Cognitive Behaviour Therapy for Chronic Fatigue Syndrome: A Randomized Controlled Trial* (UK)	60	RCT with final assessment at 12 months 16 weekly sessions of CBT and medical care or medical care alone	Karnofsky score 80 or more Functional Rating Scale improvement of employment status Number of days in bed A timed walking test Symptom Checklist Fatigue Scale HAD Scale Illness Beliefs Scale Nature of Illness Scale Coping Behaviour Scale	73% of CBT group improved compared with 27% in the medical care only group Illness beliefs and coping mechanisms changed in the CBT group CBT leads to a substantial reduction in functional impairment	CBT more effective than medical care alone in improving patients' day-to-day functioning in the medium term Collaborative rather than adversarial approach No effect in the short term Length of intervention = 16 hr
Cox and Findley (1994) *Is Chronic Fatigue Syndrome treatable in an NHS Environment?* (UK)	28	Case series retrospective audit 6 months after discharge Therapy time range, 10–30 hr	Non-standard questionnaire	57% of the inpatients perceived themselves to be improved 6 months following discharge from an inpatient programme of CBT and graded activity	Inpatient treatment appears to benefit some patients Not RCT

(contd)

Table 5.1 (contd)

Authors and title	Subject Nos	Type of study and length of follow up	Outcome measures	Results of trial	Conclusions	Limitations of the study
Lloyd et al. (1993) *Immunologic and Psychologic Therapy for Patients with Chronic Fatigue Syndrome: A Double-blind, Placebo-controlled Trial* (Australia)	90	Double blind RCT with placebo Length 7 months Dialysable leukocyte extract and CBT or clinic Placebo and CBT or clinic CBT = 6 sessions Therapy time 3½ to 6 hr or 8 injections	Global well-being measure Physical Capacity Scale Karnofsky Performance Scale Profile of Mood States Blood T-cell subset analysis delayed type hypersensitivity test	All 4 treatment groups had a similar outcome DLE and CBT recorded greater improvement in the quality of life score	Although the benefit from CBT was no greater than from non-specific treatment, it is possible that a more intensive inpatient rehabilitation programme emphasizing increased levels of non-sedentary activity with careful supervision of measured physical goals may provide significant benefit	One single measure of functional impairment No mention of use of rest Inadequate number of sessions
Butler et al. (1991) *Cognitive Behaviour Therapy in Chronic Fatigue Syndrome* (UK)	50	Open uncontrolled case series trial with follow up at 3 months Therapy time Range 2–20 hr	Beck Depression Inventory General Health Questionnaire HAD Scale Modified Somatic Discomforts Q Fear Questionnaire Fatigue Scale Visual Analogue Scale	Overall self-rated percentage improvement in disability of 60%. 70% described themselves as better or much better 5 patients withdrew	Suggested advice offered to patients to avoid physical and mental activity is counterproductive Therapy led to substantial	Not RCT therefore interpret cautiously

Study	n	Design	Outcome measures	Results	Comments
See follow-up study below		26 seen as outpatients 6 seen as inpatients admission range 3–6 weeks	Problems and Targets Scale Outcome Scale	improvements in overall disability, fatigue, somatic and psychiatric symptoms	
Bonner et al. (1994) Chronic Fatigue Syndrome: A Follow-up Study (UK)	46(29)	Postal and interview survey 4 years following previous study	Fatigue Scale (modified) General Health Questionnaire HAD Scale At interview; SADS Beck Depression Inventory Modified Somatic Discomforts Questionnaire Visual Analogue Scale Self-rated global improvement	Improvement was sustained in 14/17 who completed treatment	Patients who continue to fulfil the criteria for CFS 4 years after diagnosis are likely to have more somatic disorders, to have been more fatigued and to have a previous psychiatric history when initially diagnosed Number followed up smaller than the original study Initial study not RCT
Simons et al. (1986) Cognitive Therapy and Pharmacology for Depression (USA)	70	Clinical trial 4 treatments CT; n = 19 TCA; n = 16 CT and placebo n = 17 CT and TCA n = 18 12-week course Follow up, 12 weeks, 1, 6 and 12 months	Beck Depression Inventory Zung Anxiety Scale Dysfunctional Attitudes Scale Automatic Thoughts Questionnaire Self-control Schedule Social Adjustment Scale Hopelessness Scale	44/70 responded to treatment 28/44 remained well at 1 year CT 10/19 = 53% TCA 9/19 = 56% CT and P, 11/17 = 65% CT and TCA, 14/18 = 78%	Discontinuation of TCA at 3 months not common practice Patients who received CT (with or without tricyclic antidepressants) were less likely to relapse in the 1-year follow-up period than those receiving pharmacotherapy Naturalistic design

(contd)

Table 5.1 (contd)

Authors and title	Subject Nos	Type of study and length of follow up	Outcome measures	Results of trial	Conclusions	Limitations of the study
Williams et al. (1993) *Evaluation of a Cognitive Behavioural Programme for Rehabilitating Patients with Chronic Pain* (UK)	212	Prospective longitudinal study pre-treatment end of treatment 1- and 6-month follow up 4-week inpatient programme	Sickness Impact Profile Beck Depression Inventory Pain Self-efficacy Questionnaire Walking speed and distance Pain Severity and Distress Scale Programme Satisfaction Scale	Improvements in mean scores for dysfunction, depression, self-efficacy and physical measures at treatment end, 1- and 6-month follow up	Assessment after treatment revealed significant improvements that were maintained at 6-months follow up	Not RCT, no control group Difficult to generalize

RCT = randomised controlled trial
CBT = cognitive behaviour therapy
CFS = chronic fatigue syndrome
HAD = Hospital Anxiety and Depession Scale
DLE = dialyzable leukocyte extract
SADS = Schedule for affective disorder and schizophrenia
CT = Cognitive Therapy
TCA = tricyclic antidepressants

environmental and physiological effects. Patients' current attitudes and beliefs are examined and they are assisted to discover the most useful ways of managing and overcoming their illness, by identifying how the illness affects their thoughts, feelings and behaviours (Sharpe, 1991).

A number of strategies are used to challenge and change any identified dysfunctional thinking styles. The therapist and patient work together to plan strategies to deal with clearly identified problems and emphasis is placed on self-help (Sharpe, 1991). Goals or steps are established that concentrate on an individual's major difficulties. The purpose of these goals is to facilitate:

(1) a gradual increase in tolerance to activity;
(2) a reduction in symptoms;
(3) an increase in previously avoided behaviours and activities
    (Cox, 1999a).

Conceptualism follows assessment to lead to a therapy plan (Chalder, 1997; Sharpe et al., 1997). As stated previously, therapy time is restricted often to between 10 and 16 sessions. Therapy continues between sessions with homework assignments to monitor and challenge specific thinking patterns and to implement behavioural change (Enright, 1997).

The following case vignette aims to illustrate the cognitive aspects seen within the illness.

Case Vignette 2

Phillip (aged 36) described the onset of his illness as starting shortly after splitting up from his wife $4^1/_2$ years ago. He stated this was a particularly stressful time in his life and he noted after the split that he suffered with stomach pains. He went to his GP who diagnosed anxiety and stress. These symptoms eventually went. However six months later he suffered with 'flu' and was acutely unwell for approximately two weeks. Since this time he has felt generally unwell and described his current symptoms as aches in his arms, neck and head, pain at times, a general lack of energy, nausea, anxiety, low mood and poor sleep.

Phillip described good and bad days, stating he could do very little on a bad day, apart from wash and dress. On a good day or 'average' day he stated he was able to manage work and occasionally socialize. He stated that he is currently employed in the motor trade, although in general has to have one to three months off intermittently each year. He said that to date his company has been supportive, but he expressed concern about the amount of sick leave he had had to take over the last four years. Phillip lives alone in his own house and stated that although he can work, his domestic chores are generally completed by his mother and his ex-wife. His previous hobbies were going to the gym, playing football and rugby and going to the pub with friends. He said that he still occasionally goes to the pub, but suffers for days afterwards. Phillip has previously tried amitriptyline and Prozac but stated he could not cope with the sideeffects and was currently on no medication. He stated that he has tried counselling in the past but found it difficult. Phillip's reason for attending the occupational therapy session was for some 'light at the end of the tunnel'.

Chapter 6
Graded Exercise

Graded exercise has been suggested in the management of chronic fatigue syndrome (CFS), as patients with CFS are less active than healthy people, and have been found to have an increased heart-rate response to exercise compared with sedentary but healthy controls (Fulcher and White, 1996). In addition, patients generally complain of exercise intolerance and weakness, which may be related to physical deconditioning (Fulcher and White, 1998).

Rationale for the Use of Graded Exercise in CFS

CFS is characterized by:

* unexplained weakness;
* lethargy;
* prolonged fatigue after exercise or minimal effort (Holmes et al., 1988; Fukuda et al., 1994).

Early studies of aerobic work capacity on patients with CFS concluded that patients had a reduced aerobic work capacity, and an altered perception of their degree of exertion and pre-morbid level of physical activity (Riley et al., 1990).

A large proportion of patients with CFS report a high level of activity prior to the illness and indicate an aspiration to return to previous levels of activity (Riley et al., 1990; Surawy et al., 1995). Rowbottom and colleagues (1998) supported this finding by observing low aerobic capacity in CFS patients, which appeared to be a reflection of their sedentary lifestyles necessitated by the illness.

However, impaired exercise performance did not appear to relate to diminished motivation as no differences had been noted in heart rate or respiratory exchange between CFS patients and healthy controls (Riley et al., 1990; Rowbottom et al., 1998). Patients with CFS showed an impaired capacity for exercise even though they indicated an increased perception of their exertion (Riley et al., 1990). Lloyd and colleagues (1991) were unable to support the former finding and they concluded that there was no significant difference in perceived exertion between CFS patients and controls. They suggested instead that the pathophysiological abnormality responsible for the subjective fatigability must lie within the central nervous system (CNS) above the level of the motor cortex (Lloyd et al., 1991). This theory was further supported in the study by Gibson and colleagues (1993) who concluded that raised perceived exertion scores during exercise were suggestive of CNS factors limiting exercise in CFS patients. Rowbottom and colleagues (1998) concurred that CFS patients' inability to exercise to their full capacity was perhaps due to elevated perceptions of exertion or fatigue.

As patients with CFS appeared not to exercise to their full physiological capacity, it was suggested that graduated exercise programmes could be commenced without fear of damage to muscles and were unlikely to be harmful (Gibson et al., 1993; Wilson et al., 1994b). In addition, earlier studies of mitochondria in CFS patients indicated the need for therapeutic exercise to improve both the physical and mental well-being of patients (Wagenmakers et al., 1988). However, the emphasis was placed on a graduated activity programme following adequate explanation and education rather than exercise *per se* (Peel, 1988; Denman, 1990; Wilson et al., 1994b), as patients had a tendency to return to activity too quickly and therefore exacerbate symptoms (Wilson et al., 1994b). Consequently, once an exacerbation of symptoms following activity or exercise had been experienced, patients tended to avoid or reduce their habitual activity, which if sustained led to the cycle of deconditioning (Ray et al., 1995; Clements et al., 1997). This phenomena is also seen in fibromyalgia (Bennett, 1989), a condition of unknown aetiology with a similar presentation to CFS (Buchwald and Garrity, 1994). It has been suggested that 'aggressive exercise therapy may be as unhelpful as aggressive rest therapy' (Sharpe and Wessely, 1998, p. 796).

However, the positive effects of supervised cardiovascular fitness training programmes have been reported in patients with fibromyalgia (McCain et al., 1988; Klug et al., 1989). Physical exercise appeared to improve mental status, patient global assessment scores and lead to an improvement in pain threshold, although the reduced levels of psychological distress observed were felt to be a result of socialization within the group setting rather than the exercise (McCain et al., 1988).

An interesting point from the study by McCain and colleagues (1988) was the initial deterioration in ability owing to post-exertional pain and stiffness. They emphasize the need for appropriate supervision to maintain compliance (McCain et al., 1988). This is further illustrated by Sharpe and colleagues (1997), who state that 'patients will need to be warned that the resumption of activity is likely to lead to some initial discomfort', and that such a warning should be 'accompanied by an explanation of the physiological basis of such symptoms' (p. 194). Poor compliance rates often relate to doing 'too much too soon', resulting in discomfort and possible injury even in the normal population (Klug et al., 1989, p. 36).

CFS patients often report a 'relapse' of severe symptoms in CFS after exercise which appears to be delayed, starting six to 48 hours after the exercise, and can last from two days to two weeks (McCully et al., 1996). Delayed fatigue and muscle pain are well recognized physiological phenomena that usually occur between 24 and 48 hours after any exertion in excess of a person's current fitness (Joyce and Wessely, 1996). McCully and colleagues (1996) noted that a variety of different exercise routines from mild to strenuous activity have been used in studies, with patients following mild exercise routines not necessarily experiencing relapses. They concluded that the intensity of the exercise, the immune response and/or the psychological stress associated with the exercise could induce a relapse rather than the exercise alone (McCully et al., 1996). This finding again indicates the importance of careful explanation and guidance when commencing exercise or activity (Sharpe et al., 1997).

A recent randomized controlled trial of graded exercise supported the use of appropriately prescribed graded aerobic exercise in the management of CFS (Fulcher and White, 1997), the key aspect being that exercise was prescribed and graded. The physiological and perceptual improvements seen occurred at the sub-maximal stages of exercise, which Fulcher and White (1997) noted were clinically significant. Sub-maximal activities such as walking were functionally more important than maximal activities such as running (Fulcher and White, 1997). Interestingly, although more patients rated themselves as functionally better in this and a previous study (McCain et al., 1988), the exercise did not improve mood or sleep. This perhaps suggests that these aspects need to be treated prior to commencing an exercise programme.

Graded exercise in the treatment of CFS appears to be useful (Fulcher and White, 1997, 1998). The evidence indicates that patients with CFS should not simply be encouraged to increase their activity level. Therefore, the cognitive processes that lie at the root of their physical inactivity, such as attributing the illness to a physical cause and/or believing that activity is harmful and leads to fatigue, need to be addressed (Chalder, Power and Wessely, 1996; Vercoulen et al., 1997).

The Practice of Graded Exercise

The terms exercise and activity are often used interchangeably (Sharpe et al., 1997). In the main, most clinicians and therapists advocate a gradual increase in daily activities rather than specific exercise (Wilson et al., 1994b; Sharpe et al., 1997). However, it has been suggested that a graded increase in activity is unlikely to be effective unless associated psychological factors are attended to (Wilson et al., 1994b).

The types of exercise found to be beneficial in fibromyalgia were swimming, cycling, jogging, walking or rowing. These activities all primarily employ large muscle groups (Klug et al., 1989), the main requirement is that exercise should elicit a sustained increase in heart rate, to enhance cardiovascular fitness (Klug et al., 1989).

The types of exercise and activities prescribed for CFS patients should be adapted to their current capability, and goals set that are realistic, achievable and increased in a step-wise manner (Fulcher and White, 1998; Cox, 1999a). It is recommended that sessions should be carried out by a qualified exercise therapist, and supported by written instructions. Exercise intensity and duration should be adapted for the individual and progress determined by response (McCully et al., 1996; Fulcher and White, 1998).

The initial aim is to establish a regular pattern of exercise, usually walking, for a small amount per day such as five minutes, with the exercise session scheduled into the daily routine of activity and rest (Sharpe et al., 1997; Fulcher and White, 1998; Cox, 1999a). Exercise target heart rates are calculated for each patient and monitored throughout treatment to assess cardiovascular response (McCully et al., 1996; Fulcher and White, 1998). The type of exercise is increased in duration and/or intensity as improvement is noted (Fulcher and White, 1998).

The most important aspects of an exercise programme are consistency and grading (Royal Colleges, 1996; Sharpe et al., 1997; Cox, 1999a). Patients need to be encouraged not to over-exert themselves in an attempt to speed up the recovery process, as this could lead to a severe exacerbation of symptoms and consequent avoidance of future activity or exercise (Joyce and Wessely, 1996; Royal Colleges, 1996). The overall aim of a rehabilitation programme, of which exercise forms a part, is to place the patient back in control of the symptoms rather than the symptoms controlling the patient (Sharpe et al., 1997; Cox, 1999a).

The following case vignette aims to illustrate an onset, presentation and an attempt at self-directed management of the illness, with the use of exercise.

Case Vignette 3

Fiona (aged 48) described her illness as starting six years ago following a 'flu-like' illness from which she felt she never recovered. She described her current symptoms on attendance at the occupational therapy initial session as extreme tiredness, daily headache, general weakness, aching neck, sensitivity to light and tinnitus. She stated that at the onset of the illness she had been unable to keep her balance. At times she had collapsed and been taken to her local hospital for investigations but no cause for her symptoms had been identified.

Fiona said she lived with her husband and two children aged 14 and 16 in their own house. She said she could manage her own self-care but needed her husband's assistance with domestic chores, especially the shopping. She could walk indoors but needed a wheelchair outdoors. At the onset of the illness Fiona was a librarian; she had not worked since the onset. Fiona stated that she had experienced a number of stressful events in the last 10 years, these being: a car crash, a number of bereavements, moving house and undergoing a hysterectomy nine years ago.

She stated that she had recently been started on 20 mg of amitriptyline two hours prior to bed at night and though this assisted with getting off to sleep, she was still waking frequently during the night. On waking in the morning she did not feel refreshed.

She said she had previously enjoyed gardening and attempted to do gentle exercises at home, but often overdid it and would need to rest for a number of days before attempting to recommence her exercise routine. Her reason for attendance at the occupational therapy session was to learn as much as possible.

Chapter 7
Occupational Therapy and Lifestyle Management

To support someone with chronic fatigue sundrome (CFS), consideration of all aspects of daily life and the interaction of behaviour, emotion, symptoms and thoughts are required (Surawy et al., 1995). In 1994, the College of Occupational Therapists (COT) issued a position statement on core skills and the conceptual foundation for the practice of occupational therapy and defined the task of an occupational therapist (OT) as follows:

> The OT assesses the physical, psychological and social functions of the individual, identifies areas of dysfunction and involves the individual in a structured programme of activity to overcome disability. The activities selected will relate to the consumer's personal, social, cultural and economic needs and will reflect the environmental factors which govern his life. (College of Occupational Therapists, 1994)

In the past, the dominant model of practice in medicine has been the 'biomedical' model. More recently the 'biopsychosocial' model has been suggested to overcome the limitations of the biomedical model (Engel, 1980). The biomedical model related to the mechanisms of disease rather than the individual, whereas the biopsychosocial model allows equal assessment of the biological and psychosocial aspects of a patient (Royal Colleges, 1996), therefore enabling a more comprehensive picture of the individual. As can be seen from the COT definition (1994), an OT's assessment is based within a biopsychosocial framework, as the OT assesses all aspects of the individual that might result in dysfunction.

A biopyschosocial approach has been recommended in the assessment and treatment of CFS (Yeomans and Conway, 1991; Royal Colleges, 1996), although it has been suggested that this method might prove difficult to implement in practice as few physicians have been properly trained in the approach (Straus, 1996). However, OTs have been trained in such an approach and therefore are well suited to assist in the management of CFS (Pemberton et al., 1994; Essame et al., 1998; Cox, 1999a).

The term 'lifestyle management' was formulated from Hagedorn's (1995) discussion on occupational balance, and the work of Wilson and colleagues (1994b) who suggested the term when summarizing the management of CFS thus:

> The symptomatic treatment of sleep disturbance, pain, and concurrent psychologic morbidity (pharmacologically or psychologically), together with simple advice on lifestyle management and avoidance of factors that may potentiate the disability, would appear sound practice. (p. 548)

It has been suggested that occupational integration of form and performance can be achieved by the use of therapeutic intervention promoting lifestyle change (Lambert, 1998). The occupational form is the thing that is done and the occupational performance is the doing (Nelson, 1997). This forms the basis of occupations theory in occupational therapy (Christiansen and Baum, 1997a; Creek, 1997a). Christiansen and Baum (1997a) have taken this concept further and have stated that:

> ...occupations are human pursuits that are: goal directed and purposeful; performed in situations or contexts that influence them; can be identified by the doer and others; and are meaningful. (p. 7)

The terms function and occupational performance are often used synonymously, function referring to an individual's performance of activities, tasks and roles during daily living occupations (occupational performance) (Ottenbacher and Christiansen, 1997).

Lifestyle has been defined by Lambert (1998) as:

> ...the pattern of life adopted by an individual, or group, which is influenced by the resources available to them...specific elements include, diet, physical activity, rest, habits, routines, and social interactions in which they participate regularly. (p. 194)

Therefore the term 'Occupational Therapy Lifestyle Management' encompasses the principles and processes of occupations theory and the need to reformulate lifestyle behavioural patterns to enable management of CFS by a structured programme of activity (COT, 1994; Wilson et al., 1994b; Wessely, 1995c; Fulcher and White, 1997; Cox, 1999a).

Historical Context of Occupational Therapy

Occupational therapy was pioneered in America in the late nineteenth century by a scattered group of professionals: two psychiatrists, a physician, a nurse, a teacher of design, a social worker and two architects, hence the diversity of the profession (Hagedorn, 1997; Paterson, 1997). George Barton, an architect, first coined the term 'occupational therapy' in 1914 (Hagedorn, 1995). The first school of occupational therapy in the UK was set up by Dr Elizabeth Casson, a psychiatrist, in 1930 (Hagedorn, 1995; Paterson, 1997). However, the origins of occupational therapy in the UK can be traced back to the use of work therapy in tuberculosis sanatoriums in the early 20th century (Bryder, 1987).

Hall, when discussing neurasthenia [CFS] in the USA in 1905, stated:

> ...there is nothing new in the idea that physical work is mentally and physically hygienic and that idleness of any sort is likely to breed doubts and uncertainties and worries. (p. 30)

Hall (1905) goes on to state that if the patient could be got 'to care for something outside his own little circle of troubles, at work perhaps at some absorbing occupation, a cure would be accomplished' (p. 30).

He set up a shop run by a competent teacher and assistants to make pottery items, rugs by weaving, and baskets, with neurasthenic patients introduced for a short time each day. This appears to be the basis of graded activity principles and occupation to assist recovery in CFS. He advocated a very gradual progressive programme, which was written out and entrusted to a nurse to ensure it was carried out as written. The hours of rest were gradually made shorter and the hours of work longer (Hall, 1905).

From the work within the asylums in the 19th century and early 20th century, the occupational therapy profession in Britain developed in all areas of health care (Paterson, 1997). Much of the profession's history in the UK is associated with the creation of the National Health Service (NHS) in 1948 (Paterson, 1998). The advances in medical science and technology such as prevention by vaccines and the treatment by antibiotics of such illnesses as tuberculosis and poliomyelitis have transformed health care and consequently have had an impact on occupational therapy. In particular, the length of time needed for healing and rehabilitation has greatly reduced, in both the psychiatric and physical fields, due to improved techniques and effective therapy (Paterson, 1998). However, these improvements have enabled a greater number of people to reach old age and have necessitated an expansion of services to meet the demand for assessment and rehabilitation (Paterson, 1998).

Occupational therapists now work in all areas of health and the life spectrum (Paterson, 1998). Occupational therapy practice has widened from the NHS into many areas including social services, schools, private hospitals and practice, industry, prisons and general practice, indicating the importance of the profession in enabling occupation in all areas of life (Paterson, 1997, 1998).

Theoretical Foundations of Occupational Therapy

Christiansen and Baum (1997a) have stated that 'occupations are performed by persons in environments', thus three elements – persons, environments and occupational performance – were used to conceptualize a model of occupational therapy: the Person–Environment–Occupational Performance Model (p. 20). The Person–Environment–Occupational Performance model is client centred, as it focuses on the individual and that person's daily occupations which are limited as the result of a health condition or disability (Rogers, 1951; CAOT, 1991; Christiansen and Baum, 1997b).

Occupational performance is:

> ...the product of the dynamic relationship among persons, their occupations and roles, and the environment in which they live, work and play. (Law et al., 1997, p. 74)

There are many theoretical models of practice in occupational therapy that have emerged based on the person–environment–occupation relationship. The person–environment–occupation model as described by Law and colleagues (1997) builds upon previous work (CAOT, 1991), its basis being that the occupational therapy intervention offers multiple pathways for eliciting change to enable optimal occupational performance in occupations defined as important by the client (Law et al., 1997). The person's values and daily dilemmas are incorporated into the occupational therapy intervention. This is the foundation for occupational therapy management in CFS (see Chapters 5 and 6). The authors (Law et al., 1997) are aware that the model has its limitations, as it has had limited testing and only includes minimal information on roles and their relationship with persons and occupation.

The terms 'occupation' and 'activity' are often used interchangeably (Creek, 1997a; Golledge, 1998a). Creek (1997a) defines activity as 'the performance by an individual for a specific purpose on a particular occasion' and occupation as 'a sphere of action over a period of time that is perceived by the individual as part of their social identity' (p. 33). Creek (1997a) goes on to state that 'occupation has meaning for the individual and forms part of their personal framework'.

Wilcox (1998) defined occupation as:

[the] synthesis of doing, being and becoming which is engaged in not only by individuals but also at community, national and international levels for cultural, social and political purposes. (p.341)

Occupation is thus the central aspect of human experience and an important determinant of health and well-being (Wilcox, 1998).

The theoretical foundations of occupational therapy therefore lie in the construct that people need to engage in purposeful activity to enhance health and well being (Hagedorn, 1995; Creek, 1997a; Law et al., 1997). The philosophical base of occupational therapy is derived from various frames of reference, models for practice, constraints and demands, and techniques and strategies for intervention (Creek, 1997a). A precise paradigm for the profession has not yet been universally agreed and is therefore still in development (Creek, 1997a). However, certain theories have been organized into frames of reference such as biomechanical, neurodevelopmental, rehabilitation and cognitive perceptual for physiological practice, and biological, psychodynamic, humanistic, behavioural and cognitive for psychological practice (Creek, 1997b; Hagedorn, 1997).

There are many overlaps between the frames of reference and therapists will often alternate between them dependent on the patient's need (Hagedorn, 1997). The physiological frames of reference tend to depend on the therapist deciding on the intervention and the patient participating, actively or passively, whereas the psychological frames of reference tend to involve the patient and the therapist working together with the therapist in a facilitator role (Creek, 1997b; Hagedorn, 1997). Occupational therapists often use an eclectic approach combining physiological and psychological frames of reference dependent on patient need (Kelly, 1995; Chevalier, 1997). The diversity in philosophical outlook being indicative of a dynamic profession in a rapidly changing world (Chevalier, 1997; Creek, 1997a).

In the management of CFS, a combination of physiological and psychological frames of reference has been used (Pemberton et al., 1994; Wilson et al., 1994b; Surawy et al., 1995; Fulcher and White, 1996; Essame et al., 1998; Cox, 1999a). Occupational therapy being involved in structured goal setting, time management, graded exposure to activity (occupations), relaxation therapy, and supportive counselling within a client-centred biopsychosocial framework (CAOT, 1991; Cox and Findley, 1994, 1998; Pemberton et al., 1994; Essame et al., 1998; Cox, 1998, 1999a). The aim is to modify occupational performance towards a comprehensive change in lifestyle with an increase in the individual's level of ability, reduced symptoms and a positive change in thinking style and management of the illness (Pemberton et al., 1994; Cox, 1999a). As previously discussed (see Chapter 6) the goal of therapy is to provide the patients with internal control to alter their behaviour (occupations).

The Practice of Occupational Therapy

Occupational therapists treat the person for whom the consequences of the disease or injury has disrupted their ability to participate in everyday activities (Fleming, 1994). It has been suggested that physicians are concerned with the cause of disease and OTs with the consequences, focusing on an individual's abilities rather than disabilities (Fleming, 1994). OTs, by retraining or teaching everyday life tasks, help a person to reconstruct a meaningful life, the basis of which is placed within a biopsychosocial context as:

- daily tasks are performed by the biological self;
- motivated by the psychological self;
- assessed by the social self.

OTs therefore design programmes to help bring about the desired change based on the probable biological, psychological or social causes of functional limitations (COT, 1994; Fleming, 1994).

OTs have a unique perspective on the relationship between function and occupation (Golledge, 1998b). Golledge (1998a) describes occupations as 'the daily living tasks that are part of an individual's lifestyle' (p. 102).

The use of occupations is fundamental to the practice of occupational therapy, both as the major goal of intervention and as the main tool to bring about change (Creek, 1997b; Golledge, 1998a).

The patient chooses occupations to use in therapy that are meaningful and purposeful for him/her as an individual (Christiansen and Baum, 1997a; Golledge, 1998a). Occupational therapy therefore fundamentally enables individuals to cope with the tasks of everyday life. These tasks may not always be physical, but may be cognitive, emotional and/or spiritual (Golledge, 1998c), the important aspect being the consistency and grading of the chosen occupations (activities/tasks) (Royal Colleges, 1996; Sharpe et al., 1997; Cox, 1999a).

The theory of occupational performance fits well with the cognitive behavioural model previously discussed (see Chapters 1 and 5), as what we do affects our feelings and thoughts as much as what we think and feel affects what we do. In addition, the principle of cognitive behaviour therapy to resume activity using clearly defined, modest and predictable goals is also the basis of occupational therapy.

Whilst the current section has described the management and treatment utilized in CFS, Section Four will go on to discuss a CFS service from its development by the author, and the specific occupational therapy approach. The following case vignette aims to illustrate an onset and presentation of the illness for a patient who was admitted as an inpatient.

Case Vignette 4

Michael (aged 25), on inpatient admission to the CFS service, was unable to tolerate any sound or light and required assistance in all areas of daily life. He had been predominantly in bed at home for two years prior to admission, only able to transfer to the wheelchair to go to the toilet two to three times a day. His mother had given up her job as a secretary to care for Michael full time. Conversation was limited to short five- to 10-minute sessions two to three times a day. Michael described a disturbed sleep pattern, at times sleeping during the day and being awake at night, or continuously catnapping, with no deep or extended sleep. On observation Michael was extremely thin, as he found it difficult to eat enough to sustain his weight due to the energy chewing and swallowing took.

Over a period of time it was possible to gain a history of the illness from Michael and his parents. The illness had started four years previously when Michael was in his final year of university. Michael did not recall a specific illness at the outset but described feeling increasingly tired throughout his third year at university, and he eventually had to go home. He was unable to return to university to complete his studies. He had attempted to restart activity prior to admission but stated that he never seemed to get beyond a certain point and he always relapsed after some weeks. He said it would then take weeks or months to regain his previous level (which was never more than being able to transfer and wash and feed himself).

Prior to admission Michael's illness dominated the house; his mother no longer used the vacuum cleaner or mowed the lawn, in an attempt to limit noise, and had the curtains in the house permanently drawn to restrict light.

Section Four:
The Occupational Therapy Approach

This service and the specific occupational therapy approach developed as a result of the interest of the author while she was a senior occupational therapist working on a neurosciences unit of a south-east England general hospital from 1988 to 1998. The main aspects of development were that it was based on the resources available and patient need. The author was also often asked about how to set up a service. The particular service is therefore described to illustrate one approach to the development and establishment of a service for patients with chronic fatigue syndrome.

Chapter 8
The Chronic Fatigue Syndrome Service

Background to Approach and Service Development

In 1990, one of the unit's neurologists started to admit patients with fatigue of unknown origin. Initially the patients were assessed by the occupational therapist (OT) alongside the general neurological caseload. The occupational therapist was asked to carry out comprehensive functional assessments to assist in deciding how much the fatigue disturbed the patients' daily lives (Cox, 1999a). During the two years following 1990 there was a gradual increase in the number of people with fatigue seen by the consultant through the medical outpatient clinics at the hospital (Cox, 1998). Many patients required inpatient admission to:

(1) confirm diagnosis through history and clinical evaluation;
(2) commence appropriate medication;
(3) commence the education into management of the illness.

Between 1991 and 1994 an investigation was carried out into the types of treatments offered to these patients in the UK (Wessely, 1989, 1990, 1991, 1992; Sharpe, 1991). In 1992, three beds were allocated within the neurology unit specifically for chronic fatigue syndrome (CFS) patients, using staffing resources already in place. During 1992 and 1993 the treatment and management approach was developed and adapted by the author as new ideas, techniques and theories were learnt (Cox and Findley, 1994; Cox, 1998).

From 1990 to 1992, 50 patients with fatigue were seen as inpatients. Twenty-eight of those patients who fulfilled the Center for Disease Control (CDC) criteria (Holmes et al., 1988) for CFS were audited (Cox and Findley, 1994), and 57% ($n = 16$) stated that they had an increased activity level six months following discharge. In February 1993, the initial protocol for admission to the unit was written. Interest and enthusiasm in treating the illness developed as patients made consistent progress that continued on their return home (Cox and Findley, 1994). Since July 1994 the service has been managed as a separate service, within the neurosciences directorate of the hospital. The inpatient beds had increased to six dedicated beds by April 1995, with an increase in nursing establishment to reflect the increased workload (Cox, 1998).

From 1995 to 1997 the therapy team staff increased to four full-time OTs, a senior physiotherapist and two part-time (18 hours) counsellors, for the inpatient and outpatient services, supported by medical and nursing staff. An A&C grade III clerical post was established to assist with the administration of the service. All the team and auxiliary staff were educated by the OTs in the principles of cognitive behaviour therapy (CBT) and the process of management.

A further audit in May 1996 indicated that 82% of patients had a perceived improved activity level at six months following discharge (Cox and Findley, 1998). It is the previous audit findings that prompted the commencement of an inpatient controlled trial. The results of this trial are awaiting publication. However, a significant effect was shown in the patients' perceived health, length of time tired, and management of the illness, as 72% of the inpatient group, compared with 44% of the comparison group, stated that they felt better than the previous year and indicated better management of their illness. These findings give some evidence of the need for an inpatient CFS management programme for specific patients with complex CFS (Cox, 1999b).

The CFS Service is a national service for outpatients and inpatients. It functions as a multidisciplinary specialist team, led and governed by the fundamental principle of Occupational Therapy and Lifestyle Management (see Chapter 7) using grading and balancing of daily activity, capitalizing on the theory of CBT (see Chapter 5), following normal clinical assessment (see Chapter 3; Cox, 1999a).

Levels of Ability

Patients with CFS can present with a wide range of symptoms and levels of ability. For ease of identifying the type of management approach required, the patients referred to the hospital are divided into four levels of ability. The levels were devised so that each patient is categorized dependent upon level of fatigue, daily activity level and general mobility (Cox, 1998; Cox and Findley, 1998):

* Mild (Grade 1)
* Moderate (Grade 2)

* Severe (Grade 3)
* Very severe (Grade 4)

- The patients in the *mild* category will be mobile and self-caring and able to manage light domestic and work tasks with extreme difficulty. The majority will still be working. However, in order to remain in work they will have stopped all leisure and social pursuits, often taking days off. Most will use the weekend to rest in order to cope with the week.
- The patients in the *moderate* category will have reduced mobility and be extremely restricted in all activities of daily living, often having peaks and troughs of ability, dependent on the degree of symptoms. The patients in this group have usually stopped work and require many rest periods, often sleeping in the afternoon for one to two hours. Sleep quality at night is generally poor and disturbed. This level appears to be the group most cited in the description of studies and CFS services (Cox and Findley, 1994; Wilson et al., 1994b; Sharpe et al., 1996; Vercoulen et al., 1996; Deale et al., 1997; Fulcher and White, 1997).
- The patients in the *severe* category will be able to carry out minimal daily tasks only, such as face washing and cleaning teeth, have severe cognitive difficulties and be wheelchair dependent for mobility. These patients are often unable to leave the house except on rare occasions with a severe prolonged after-effect from effort.
- The patients in the *very severe* category will be unable to mobilize or carry out any daily task for themselves and are 'bed-bound' for the majority of the time. These patients are often unable to tolerate any noise, and are generally extremely sensitive to light.

Components of the CFS Service

A number of different types of intervention were developed within the service. The CFS Service offered both outpatient therapy such as OT one-to-one lifestyle management, an OT lifestyle management group, OT support package, sessional physiotherapy, sessional counselling and inpatient management (Cox, 1998, 1999a; see Figure 8.1).

Depending on the distance they needed to travel, patients in the mild to moderate categories were generally able to cope with outpatient management and therapy (Cox, 1998). It has been suggested that patients in the severe to very severe categories generally require inpatient care (Royal Colleges, 1996; Essame et al., 1998). However, travelling is for the majority of patients very difficult, as the effort involved often leaves the patient unable then to cope with an outpatient session owing to mental and physical fatigue. For some patients the mere thought of attending regular outpatient therapy sessions often precluded their attendance for fear of the after-effect (Cox, 1998). The following section will describe the process of referral and briefly describe each component of the service.

Referral Protocol

Prior to admission each patient was referred to the consultant neurologist and attended the outpatient clinic at the hospital, for provisional assessment and evaluation. The OT (s) attend the new-patient and follow-up medical clinics to support the consultant in identifying the most appropriate course of action, i.e. inpatient treatment, outpatient therapy, investigations only, monitoring through clinic, referral to other services or no action. Figure 8.1 illustrates the process of referral within the service.

Inpatient Programme

The inpatient programme has been required for 20% of the patients seen in clinic (Cox, 1999a). In order to be placed on the waiting list for admission the patient needs to fulfil the following criteria:

(1) to be one of the four categories of ability;
(2) to require commencement of appropriate medication under supervision to assist with symptoms of sleep disturbance, myalgia and head discomfort;
(3) to have a diagnosis established by thorough clinical evaluation;
(4) to be outside a reasonable travelling distance for outpatient therapy;
(5) to need to partake in an in-depth rehabilitation and management programme of graded activity and CBT, to educate in day-to-day

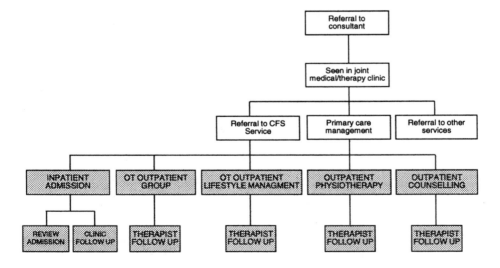

Figure 8.1 Process of referral to the CFS Service.

management, stabilize/improve daily functional ability and promote return to previous levels of ability;

(6) to need to have a change of environment, owing to total disruption of daily life, failure of family structure, or development of illness behavioural patterns;

(7) to have not responded to or coped with outpatient treatment.

The patients are admitted into one of the dedicated beds on a mixed-gender neurological ward. In the first two weeks of admission the patient is fully screened. Initially the patient is admitted by a senior house officer and the following investigations are booked:

- haematological tests: full blood count, ESR, LFT, U&E, T4, TSU, CPK;
- biochemical tests: thyroid function;
- immunological tests: auto antibody screening, total and differential immunoglobulins, circulating immune complexes, enterovirus IgG, IgM antibody, VP1 antigen and glandular fever screen;
- evoked potentials: auditory and visual;
- electroencephalogram (EEG);
- magnetic resonance imaging (MRI) scan;
- electromyograph (EMG);
- electrocardiogram (ECG);
- rheumatoid screen.

Additional tests are booked dependent upon clinical indications and may include X-rays, muscle biopsy and nerve conduction studies.

Following the investigation and exclusion of other causes, a diagnosis of CFS is made based on the criteria from the CDC in Atlanta, Georgia, USA (Fukuda et al., 1994; see Figure 1.2 and Chapter 3).

The minimum length of stay is two weeks for assessment with a maximum length of stay of up to 10 weeks. A review admission is occasionally required six months following discharge to review the patient's current level of ability, adapt the management and review medication (Cox, 1998, 1999a).

Once on the ward each patient is seen individually by a specific allocated OT for a minimum of three contact sessions per week (see Chapter 9). The time length of the session will depend on the individual's level of concentration. In general, each session ranges from half to one hour (Cox, 1998, 1999a; Cox and Findley, 1998; see Chapter 9). Patients are also referred to the CFS team physiotherapist for assessment of posture, mobility, joint and muscle function and the CFS team counsellor, if required or requested by individuals.

Occupational Therapy Group

The group is a closed group for patients in the mild to moderate categories who require in-depth information. The aim of the group is to enable adaptation and management of lifestyle, and improvement of daily functional ability through educational talks, discussion, role-play and demonstration. It runs for eight weeks with a maximum of eight patients, co-facilitated by two OTs. Seven weeks are concurrent, and the eighth week is two to three months following completion of the group as a follow-up review session (Cox, 1998). Before commencing the group each patient has an individual interview as described in Chapter 9.

The topics for each week are as follows:

Week One   What is CFS?
Week Two   Balance and Baselines
Week Three Rest and Relaxation
Week Four   Pacing and Grading
Week Five   Goal Planning and Anxiety Management
Week Six   Emotions and Feelings
Week Seven The Way Forward

One of the benefits of the group is that people are mixing with others who have CFS, often for the first time, and, in particular, learning from others' experiences. Frequently, after completion of the group the members will continue to act as a support network for one another. The types of comments patients have made at the end of the group are:

> I feel more in control of my life.
> I have better management of my energy.
> I gained support from others. It was great to know I wasn't the only one suffering this illness.

Occupational Therapy Lifestyle Management Consultation

This is an individual two-hour consultation for patients in the mild to moderate categories. The aim is to educate the patient and his/her signifi-cant other(s) in the principles of daily management. An extensive initial interview with the patient is carried out as part of the session (see Chapter 9). This is followed by an introduction to the topic areas of the next seven sessions described in Chapter 9. Specifically, patients are introduced to the patterns that can influence ability, and suggestions for future manage-ment are made. Follow up and review are offered as required by the patient either by telephone, letter and/or face to face, for further adapta-tion or modification of the management approach.

Outpatient Physiotherapy

Between six and 12 sessions are offered to patients with predominant symptoms of pain and/or daily headache.

Outpatient Counselling

Ten counselling sessions are offered to patients, if required and at their request.

The following chapter will describe the specific aspects of occupational therapy in CFS management.

Chapter 9
Occupational Therapy Lifestyle Management Programme

Occupational therapists (OTs) have much to offer in the management of chronic fatigue syndrome (CFS). Treatment of CFS with cognitive behaviour therapy (CBT) has previously been carried out by psychiatrists, psychologists and specialist nurse practitioners (Butler et al., 1991; Lloyd et al., 1993; Sharpe et al., 1996; Deale et al., 1997). The occupational therapy programme to be described was developed based on patients' needs and clinical presentation over the last 10 years (Cox, 1999a). A recent pilot study of inpatients (Essame et al., 1998) and a previous study of outpatients (Pemberton et al., 1994) indicated the importance of occupational therapy with this group of patients.

The Lifestyle Management Programme is based on occupational therapy theory and encompasses the biopsychosocial model (Engel, 1980; Christiansen and Baum, 1997b; Sharpe et al., 1997). The programme uses the principles of CBT (Sharpe, 1991) and graded activity (Sharpe et al., 1997; Cox and Findley, 1998). Sharpe (1998) has stated that 'CBT requires a skilled therapist, and few such therapists are available' (p. 61).

To ensure a consistent approach in the use of CBT principles within the occupational therapy programme, all OTs on the CFS team completed formal training in CBT.

As the programme has developed it is now apparent that it falls within the Canadian Occupational Performance Model guidelines for client-centred practice (CAOT, 1991; Law et al., 1997), although at the time it was developed this model was unknown. The client-centred approach encourages patients to direct their own therapy, to accept personal responsibility and to make decisions (Rogers, 1951; CAOT, 1991). In practice, the OT must address certain questions in order to gain an understanding of the factors necessary to enable function and well-being, as each patient's needs will be unique (Christiansen and Baum, 1997a).

The OT acts as a facilitator, offering opportunities and education, enabling the patients to explore thoughts and feelings in a safe therapeutic environment (CAOT, 1991; Cox and Findley, 1994, 1998; see Appendices 2 and 3). This is the basis of CBT (Sharpe et al., 1997; Cox and Findley, 1998). The main emphasis of the CFS occupational therapy programme is dealing with problems identified by the patient, and using activities that are meaningful to the individual (Christiansen and Baum, 1997a). The aim following intervention is for the patient to have an increase in his/her level of ability, reduced symptoms and a positive change in thinking style and management of the illness.

The intervention is an approach (programme) or series of 10 educational topics for daily management of CFS. These are:

(1) initial interview (assessment);
(2) daily activity level;
(3) rest and relaxation;
(4) graded activity;
(5) reintroduction of activity;
(6) exercise and sleep patterns;
(7) feelings and thoughts;
(8) coping with others;
(9) planning for home;
(10) conclusions and the future.

Assessment

Initial Interview (Session 1)

The OT carries out a specific detailed interview (see Figure 9.1) to establish:

* predisposing, precipitating and perpetuating factors;
* patient's view of cause, their own plan for recovery and purpose of admission;
* the present and past level of daily functional ability;
* present and past work capacity;
* predominant symptoms that disrupt daily life;
* previous and present rehabilitation techniques or procedures used;
* individual thoughts and feelings related to the condition and abilities.

The assessment process is essential, the most important aspect of the assessment being the taking of the full history, to identify the predisposing, precipitating and perpetuating factors and the patient's under-

Chronic Fatigue Syndrome

Initial interview

Date of interview _____ Client name _____

Checklist

- Presenting problem. Duration, frequency, severity
- Previous and current treatment. Current medication
- Domestic situation and history
- Employment situation and history
- Social contacts
- Previous traumas and any previous psychological disturbances
- Physical: exercise, appetite, sleep pattern
- Any notable medical aspects
- Consumption of alcohol, non-prescribed drugs, tobacco and caffeine
- Client's view of cause of current difficulties and any plan for their resolution
- Client's purpose in coming to see you, i.e. his/her goals

    Where do you feel you are now compared with prior to your illness (1–10)
    Where do you feel you could get to (1–10)
    How much do you feel you can influence your recovery (1–10)
    How much do you feel others can influence your recovery (1–10)

Notes: ....
....
....
....
....
....
....
....
....

Figure 9.1 Initial interview handout.

standing of the illness (Sharpe et al., 1997). Information on the patient's employment and domestic situation and history also needs to be explored to realize the full impact the illness has on the patient and his/her life.

An observational assessment of current activity levels is carried out to create a picture of daily functioning (see Figure 9.2). At the end of the interview, the patient is asked to define his/her specific aims and identify, in particular, his/her purpose for attending therapy (Sharpe et al., 1997; Cox and Findley, 1998). The report of the occupational therapy assessment is made available as required by the other team members so patients are not unnecessarily fatigued by multiple history taking.

Assessment information

Patient's name ....   Date started............................

Home situation – tick as appropriate:

	House	Council	Lease	Lift
Alone	Bungalow	Warden	Rent	Stairs (int)
Wife/husband	Bedsit	Resid.	H/sing	rail L R
	(state level)	Own	Assoc.	Stairs (ext)
	Flat (state level)		Other...........	rail L R

Other...........Heating..........Cooker — gas/elec: Access: External..........Internal..............
Community services: MOW.............. SMTWTFS   Hearing.....................
                          DN................. SMTWTFS   Sight.......................
SW.......................   HH................. SMTWTFS   Teeth......................
OT.......................   Other.............. SMTWTFS   Other.......................
Other...

Social situation/Dependants/Carers..................... Memory................................
.... Concentration.............................

Mental state/attitude	Physical state	Aids/services needed	Ordered	Supplied
Communication......................................				
Mobility/walking.....................................				
Stairs...				
Kerb/steps..				
Wheelchair...				
Other..				
Transfers: Bed......................................				
Chair.....................................				
Toilet/commode....................................				
Bath/shower...				
Other..				
PADL: washing......................................				
Dressing: Top.......................................				
Bottom...................................				
Footwear..				
Grooming...				
Eating/drinking.....................................				
Toileting/continence..............................				
Pills...				
Other..				
DADL: Make hot drink............................				
Cooking...				
Housework...				
Switches/sockets....................................				
Laundry...				
Shopping..				

Figure 9.2 Assessment information handout.

For homework, at the end of the initial interview (which for some inpatients may take place over a number of days), the patient is asked to complete a daily activity sheet to indicate the amount of activity they carry out on an 'average' day (see Figure 9.3). A patient may require more than one daily activity sheet if he/she is working or feels that he/she has a variety of days rather than a typical day.

The patient is also given Booklet One (see Appendix 1) and inpatients would be given Information Sheet 5 (see Appendix 2) to read and consider.

Introduction to the Principles of Management

Daily Activity Level (Session 2)

During this session, the OT introduces each patient to the principles of graded activity and CBT. The completed daily activity sheet is used to indicate whether a pattern of peaks and troughs is apparent in the patient's day.

> *Exercise*
> *In order to understand the use of the daily activity sheet [shown in Figure 9.3], it may be useful to complete your own daily record, and then look to see if you tend to block activities together with limited rest or 'time out' in between activities.*

A moderate patient's typical day will often look like the record shown in Figure 9.4. The diagram as shown in Figure 1.3 (p. 15) is then used to indicate the process that tends to happen in response to the symptoms experienced. That is, when patients feel well and more able they tend to do more activity in an attempt to catch up (peak); this then often pushes them over into fatigue (trough). They therefore rest, and because they have rested they feel more able and tend to increase activity again (peak) and so on. The focus of the occupational therapy programme is to break the pattern of peaks and troughs so rest and effort can be balanced in a more effective way (Fleming, 1994; Cox and Findley, 1998; Cox, 1999a). At this session(s) the importance of the balance required between rest and effort is first introduced.

For homework, the patient is asked to keep a daily diary of his/her actual activity. Booklet 2 is given to the patient to read following the session, for reinforcement of the concepts discussed (see Appendix 1). If the patient was attending for a one-to-one two-hour consultation he/she would be asked to keep the diary prior to attending for use during the session.

Date:.................................Name:..

Daily activity sheet

Time	Activity

Figure 9.3 Daily activity sheet.

6 June 1998   Jane Jones

Date:................................... Name:...

Daily activity sheet

Time	Activity
9:00 am	Get up, get washed, dressed. Have breakfast. Feed dog, make packed lunches
10:00 am–12:00 noon	Do various bits of housework
1:00 pm	Prepare and eat lunch
2:00–5:00 pm	Rest, often sleep
5:00 pm	Walk dog (sometimes)
6:00–8:00 pm	Feed children, talk to family, watch TV
9:00 pm	Go to bed

Figure 9.4 Typical moderate patient day.

The Process of Re-establishing Activity

Rest and Relaxation (Session 3)

Rest can mean different things to different people. Some patients with CFS feel that rest means sleeping or perhaps just sitting down and 'not doing anything'. Others feel that rest simply means being able to relax. Prior to becoming ill, patients may have found reading, watching television or talking to friends on the telephone a good way to unwind.

In practice, the author observed that CFS patients seemed to lose their ability to distinguish between important and unimportant sensations. Information appeared to bombard the ears and eyes resulting in '*sensory overload*' and fatigue. Patients with CFS often give the same importance to all sensations, which then compete for their attention. Management of sensory overload becomes just as important as physical management, and for some people it is the *most* important aspect of the daily management of CFS.

The relaxation sessions are designed to focus not solely on resting the body, but also on resting the mind (see Appendix 1, Booklet 3). The aim of relaxation is to achieve a state of minimal neurological (brain) activity (Cox, 1999a). Therefore, owing to the 'overactive brain' or 'sensory overload' experienced in CFS, the concept of rest often needs to be redefined. When the term 'rest' is used in the CFS occupational therapy programme it means *relaxation* (Cox, 1999a).

Rest needs to be scheduled into each day, regardless of the severity of symptoms, so that it becomes consistent and part of the patient's daily routine rather than varying depending upon symptoms (Sharpe et al., 1997; Cox and Findley, 1998). For some people it helps initially to structure each day to gain an understanding of the balance required between rest and effort.

Figure 9.5 is used to plan a structured day for the individual patient. The schedule is based on the patient's daily diary and completed daily activity sheet(s). It is important not to change the structure of the day too quickly to start with, for example; initially it helps to keep to the same times for getting up and going to bed and to balance out the previously longer afternoon rest throughout the day. In practice, it may also be found that some patients still require a one- to two-hour afternoon rest to start with until they get used to the idea of more frequent rest periods. The longer afternoon rest can then be reduced slowly over time.

Figure 9.6 shows an example of a daily timetable designed for a specific patient graded at the moderate level of ability.

Different types of relaxation are discussed and demonstrated with the patient during the session, or in specific relaxation practical sessions. In particular, the use of relaxation in the management of anxiety and panic attacks, fatigue levels and 'sensory overload' is discussed.

Chronic fatigue syndrome: daily programme schedule

Date:........................... Name:....................................

Time	Activity

Figure 9.5 Daily programme schedule.

For homework, the patient is encouraged to practice relaxation in rest periods and/or to assist with sleep at night. At the end of the session, Booklet 3 is given for reinforcement of the techniques discussed (see Appendix 1).

Graded Activity (Session 4)

In this session(s) the patient is introduced to the concept of an activity baseline, a foundation from which to build prior to reintroducing further activity into the day. An activity baseline is defined as:

> ...a comfortable level of activity that can be managed on a regular basis without experiencing an increase in symptoms. (Cox, 1999a, p. 60)

Chronic fatigue syndrome: daily programme chart

Date:......................... Name:.................................

Time	Activity
9:00 am	Wake up/activity session
10:00 am	Rest period
10:30 am	Activity session
12:00 noon	Rest period
12:30 pm	Activity session
2:30 pm	Rest period
3:30 pm	Activity session
5:30 pm	Rest period
6:00 pm	Activity session
8:00 pm	Rest period
8:30 pm	Activity session
9:30 pm	$\frac{1}{2}$ hour wind down
10:00 pm	Bed

Figure 9.6 Example of a daily activity schedule.

Patients usually need to work out their actual daily and weekly baseline over a number of weeks or even months. It is important that the patient's baseline is established before further activity is introduced, to ensure that he/she has reduced the peaks and troughs pattern, and therefore is starting to build up activity again, from a firm foundation (Cox, 1999a). Each patient is asked to complete a handout as shown in Figure 9.7.

A patient's initial baseline of activity will be somewhere between what he/she does on a good day compared with a bad day. For example, an individual may be able to manage 30 minutes of housework on a good day and nothing on a bad day. His/her initial baseline would therefore be about 10 minutes of housework daily. This would then be tried out, evaluated and modified as required, the main gauge being that he/she does not experience an increase of symptoms over time.

Chronic fatigue syndrome: baseline sheet

A *baseline of activity* is a comfortable level of activity that you can manage on a regular basis, without experiencing an increase in symptoms.

What would be your own baseline at present? ....

Figure 9.7 Baseline sheet.

In addition, when establishing their baseline for the first time, patients need to be warned that they may experience a slight increase in symptoms as their body adjusts to the new routine. If the increase in symptoms lasts longer than 48 hours, the patient may need to reduce the amount or length of some activities until no increase in symptoms is experienced.

An established baseline is therefore not necessarily achieved whilst the patient is an inpatient or during the course of the group or individual session (Cox and Findley, 1998). Patients often need ongoing support following completion of sessions, ranging from months to years, to adapt or modify the programme (Cox, 1999a).

Activity is defined as anything that stimulates or over-stimulates the brain in terms of physical, cognitive or emotional effort. Thus talking, watching television, reading and even eating are regarded as activities. In addition, different activities take different amounts of energy. Patients are shown how to divide activities up into the differing amounts of energy each activity takes to carry out, such as high, medium or low energy, using the handout shown in Figure 9.8.

Exercise
Complete the energy requirements handout for yourself. Divide the activities you listed in your daily activity sheet into the high, medium or low boxes. Then ask a colleague to do the same without looking at your responses. This will illustrate how personal an exercise this is, in that vacuuming for one person may be a low-energy activity but for another a high-energy activity.

Energy requirements

What category does the *activity* fall into?

How much energy does the *activity* cost you in terms of energy needed?

Low	
Medium	
High	

Figure 9.8 Energy requirements handout.

The purpose of energy grading patients' activities is to enable sustained and consistent activity on a daily and weekly basis. The idea is that they do not have all their high-energy activity together (peak) but that those activities are spread throughout the day and week, interspaced with medium and low-level activities, which enables a more paced use of their energy and therefore reduction in fatigue (Cox, 1999a).

When describing to patients how to balance their week, they are initially asked to complete the weekly plan as shown in Figure 9.9 at their current pre-management activity level. They are then asked to colour in the squares using:

- red for high-energy activities;
- green for medium-energy activities;
- blue for low-energy activities.

Chronic fatigue syndrome: weekly plan

Times											
Sunday											
Monday											
Tuesday											
Wednesday											
Thursday											
Friday											
Saturday											

Figure 9.9 Weekly plan handout.

At the end of the exercise the patient then has a visual display of his/her current peaks and troughs, often returning to the session with blocks of red only occasionally interspaced with blue or green. The weekly plan is then redesigned, spacing out the blocks of red where possible.

For homework, the patient is asked to write down all the activities he/she would like to do in the future for use at the next session, and if he/she has not already done so, to complete the baseline of activity and the energy requirements handouts.

Reintroduction of Activity (Session 5)

As a basis for discussion about the reintroduction of activity, the completed baseline of activity and individual aims and goals handouts as shown in Figures 9.10 and 9.11 are used. These are then discussed between the patient and OT.

Chronic fatigue syndrome: personal aims

Aims you would like to achieve

Your aim may be to reintroduce an activity you used to enjoy or to build on those abilities you have already achieved. Once you have decided what to work on, you need to consider how to achieve it.

(1) Think about what is involved in achieving your aim.
(2) Think about your present level of ability.
(3) Think about how you could make various aspects of the task easier for yourself.
....
....
....
....
....
....
....
....
....
....
....
....
....
....
....
....
....
....
....
....

Figure 9.10 Personal aims sheet.

Chronic fatigue syndrome: goals sheet

Once you have decided on your aims, the next stage is to formulate your goals. Goals need to be:

(1) realistic;
(2) achievable;
(3) specific;
(4) time managed.

Guidelines:

(1) Increase goals one at a time.
(2) Increase goals by a maximum of 15% each time.
(3) Goals must be increased slowly over time.
(4) Increase goals after a minimum of 4 days.
(5) Re-evaluate goals on a regular basis.

Not achieving goals does not make you a failure!

You will need to re-evaluate these goals. It may be that they were not realistic. It may be that something else got in the way (i.e. a virus, family upset). It may be because you were being too hard on yourself. Just adjust the goal itself or the time you set yourself to achieve it.

Date	Goal	Date to review

Figure 9.11 Goals sheet.

The goals need to be clear and specific, and set at a manageable level (Surawy et al., 1995). In order to assist the patient in a gradual reintroduction of activity, he/she is shown how to break an activity down into smaller components. For example, when *shopping for the weekly groceries*, initially the patient needs to consider what this would involve:

- walking;
- driving;
- parking;
- packing, lifting and carrying;
- concentration and attention;
- writing and following a list;
- coping with sensory stimulation, such as light, noise, people;
- time;
- managing money.

He/she may then decide initially to work on walking and concentration, or initially to attempt one aisle and return to the car, perhaps leaving his/her companion to complete the shop.

The targets to achieve are increased gradually so that the amount of activity carried out each day and/or week is built up slowly (Cox and Findley, 1998). The goals are changed and upgraded only when achieved and sustained.

For homework, the patient is asked to break an activity down into achievable stages, and indicate a time scale for each goal on the goal-setting handout.

Exercise and Sleep Patterns (Session 6)

In this session, the importance of gentle aerobic exercise, normalizing sleep patterns and the use of relaxation to assist in sleep and rest is discussed. Previous levels of exercise are discussed and the gradual reintroduction of exercise reinforced. A goal plan for the re-establishment of exercise is discussed and fitted in to the daily timetable.

For homework, the patient is asked to read Booklet 4 to further clarify the techniques and reasoning discussed (see Appendix 1), and to practise any planned exercise (activity).

Feelings and Thoughts (Session 7)

Throughout the occupational therapy sessions the feelings and thoughts associated with the illness are explored. The patient is encouraged to identify areas that may need to be changed. In particular, the OT facilitates the patient developing an awareness of the effects of emotions on lifestyle and the illness, and his/her own self-concepts and beliefs. The links between emotion and the body are explored. In addition, cognitive tasks are considered to assist in increasing concentration and attention, and are incorporated into each day. Booklet 5 (see Appendix 1) and the self-assessment form (see Figure 9.12) are used to assist in this process.

For homework, the patient is encouraged to continue grading future goals and long-term aims, and to use lists to aid memory. Individuals are

Self-assessment and self-help form

Instructions: Ideally this form should be completed *when you are feeling bad* (depressed, anxious, or whatever). If that is not possible, complete it *as soon as possible* afterwards.

(1) How are you feeling? Be as specific as you can. Rate the intensity of the feeling by giving it a number from 1 (slight) to 100 (very severe).

_____

_____

_____

_____

(2) What has triggered the way you are feeling? What time of day is it, what date? Where are you? What is happening? What is about to happen?

_____

_____

_____

_____

(3) What thoughts are in your mind? Rate the degree to which you believe these thoughts by giving them a number from 1 (slight) to 100 (absolutely certain).

_____

_____

_____

_____

(4) What would be more constructive thoughts to have? In filling in this section it may be useful to look at point 3 above and ask yourself, am I:

• putting too much emphasis on one aspect of the situation and disregarding other more positive aspects?
• jumping to conclusions?
• thinking in all-or-nothing terms?
• magnifying my failings/mistakes and minimizing my assets and achievements?
• being over-influenced by one thing that has gone wrong?
• being too ready to blame myself for something that has happened?

_____

_____

Now re-rate the intensity of your negative feeling, from 1 to 100.

©: APT, PO Box 3, Thurnby, Leicester LE7 9QN

Figure 9.12 Self-assessment form.

encouraged to complete self-assessment forms as required and to practise relaxation techniques.

Coping with Others (Session 8)

The average duration of the illness for most patients is four years (Cox and Findley, 1998; Cox, 1999) which can have a major disruption on relationships. In this session, the effect of the illness and relationships is discussed specifically, in particular to examine the changing roles now, and in the future as the patient gains in ability. The importance of informing and educating family and friends in the understanding of the illness and its management is also emphasized.

However, the effect of the illness on relationships is embedded into each contact session, as the specific content of each session depends on what aspects are important to the patient at that time. For each session the agenda is negotiated between the patient and therapist.

For homework, the patient is asked to consider his/her expectations, and any problems and solutions that have been discussed.

Planning for Home (Session 9 – inpatients only)

Future goals and discharge plans for inpatients are discussed with the patient well in advance of discharge. This enables appropriate selection, discussion and adaptation of the methods learnt and referral to other services for provision of care and/or equipment. During the session a proposed daily and weekly plan for home use, balancing high-, medium- and low-energy activities is considered (see Figures 9.5 and 9.8).

For homework, the patient is asked to read Booklet 6 (see Appendix 1) and Information Sheets 11 and 12 (see Appendix 2). It is suggested that he/she lists out any remaining questions to discuss in the final session(s), and reflects on the proposed daily and weekly plans, making changes to the plan as he/she feels appropriate.

Conclusions and the Future (Session 10)

This session covers a review of the principles of management and the coping strategies learnt. In particular:

- the need to balance rest and activity each day;
- the importance of sustaining activity prior to moving on to the new level of activity;
- the importance of a gradual reintroduction of previously avoided activity;
- the importance of identifying triggers and perpetuators;

- the ways to cope with and manage other illnesses such as viral infections;
- overview of general coping strategies learnt.

This session is usually held with the spouse, partner or family members. However, significant others are invited to attend any session if desired and agreed by the patient. The patient is always encouraged to bring a family member or friend to the individual two-hour outpatient session. Essame and colleagues (1998) found that progress appeared to be maintained when a good working relationship developed between the therapist, the patient and their carer.

Conclusion

The sessions would not always be carried out in the chronological order discussed above, as it would depend on the patient's need and his/her specific questions. However, in the main this order is covered for most patients. In the two-hour session all aspects are covered but in less depth and at greater speed.

The purpose of the session(s) is therefore to familiarize the patient:

- with the theory behind the concept;
- to start to establish a baseline of activity;
- to gain an understanding of the importance of balancing rest and effort;
- with the process of the reintroduction of activity over time.

In particular, it is important that the patient and his/her significant other(s) gain a thorough understanding of the lifestyle changes required, i.e. what they will need to do, by gaining knowledge of the strategies that change behaviour, attitudes and beliefs about CFS (Cox, 1998, 1999a).

Techniques Used

The techniques commonly used in the management programme are:

- discussion;
- collaboration;
- brainstorming;
- concept mapping;
- role play;
- demonstration;
- relaxation;

- breathing exercises;
- goal setting;
- homework;
- feedback and summary.

The specific cognitive therapy techniques that are used are:

- identification of negative automatic thoughts;
- identification of underlying beliefs;
- challenging and changing irrational and dysfunctional thought processes through:
  > exploring inference chains
  > cognitive rehearsal
  > thought switching/stopping
  > 'friend' technique
  > alternative thoughts
  > evidence for and against
  > advantages and disadvantages.

Case Studies

The four previously introduced case vignettes will now be used to illustrate the occupational therapy intervention in the various settings described in Chapter 8.

Case Study 1

Jane (aged 44) had described the onset of her illness as starting five years prior to attendance. The onset followed a simple operation at her local hospital for removal of a tooth abscess. She stated that at the time she was under a lot of personal stress and had financial worries. Her mother had died in the previous year. On attendance at the occupational therapy session, she described her current symptoms as right-sided weakness and pain, sudden draining of energy, headache, generalized fatigue and a dry mouth. She was currently taking 50 mg of amitriptyline two hours prior to going to bed to assist with sleep disturbance. However, she said she still had difficulty getting off to sleep, woke frequently during the night and generally woke each morning feeling unrefreshed.

At the time of the onset of the illness she was working as a music therapist at her local centre for children with learning difficulties. She had stopped work two years ago as a result of the illness. Jane lived alone in her own house and could currently manage all her own personal care activities. However, she was reliant on her family and friends to

complete domestic tasks, and was not currently able to socialize for
longer than 10 minutes with one person in her own home. She was not
able to maintain her normal social activities of attending the local
church and visiting family and friends.

When Jane was seen in clinic she was placed in the *moderate* level of
ability. It was therefore agreed by Jane, the consultant and the OT that a
two-hour occupational therapy lifestyle management consultation might
be the most appropriate treatment approach. She was commenced on 50
mg of amitriptyline at the outpatient clinic to assist with her difficulty in
getting off to sleep.

Jane attended the session with a close friend. Jane described her
purpose in attending the session as:

(1) To have a specific plan.
(2) To be able to make the best of what I have.
(3) To be able to do my own domestic chores rather than relying on others.
(4) To be able to return to work.

During the session Jane was introduced to the concepts of:

- the pattern of peaks and troughs;
- the importance of having a structured day, balancing rest and activity
  throughout the day;
- what is meant by rest and activity;
- the need to establish a baseline of activity, consider energy requirements and the importance of pacing activity;
- the need to reintroduce activity in a gradual and systematic way over
  time;
- the importance of having realistic and achievable goals in order to
  achieve personal aims;
- the influence of feelings and thoughts on the illness and ways of identifying, challenging and changing any recurring negative thought
  patterns;
- the effect of the illness on friends and family relationships and the
  importance of maintaining open channels of communication.

At the end of the session Jane appeared to understand the concepts and
stated that she would attempt to put the techniques discussed into
practice at home. She was unsure of how the timetable of rest and activity
would work at home but said she would 'give it a go'. Jane was encouraged to stay in touch with the OT. The set of six booklets and various
handouts were given to Jane to use as a resource.

A week after the session Jane got in touch with the OT to adjust the structured daily routine devised during the session. Jane had found on commencing the routine at home that one of the rest periods needed to be earlier. This was discussed and adjusted over the telephone for Jane to re-try. Jane at this time also discussed the goals she had set herself for restarting her own domestic chores and future work. With regard to the domestic chores, she had broken each activity down and set herself a timetable to recommence components of the tasks over time.

As far as work was concerned, she had made enquires at her local school about classroom assistant work as a volunteer. She had agreed with the head teacher that she would attempt to commence half an hour a week initially in the following winter term (six months from setting the goal).

Jane remained in contact over the following two years, at times on a weekly basis, then monthly and then sporadically.

She is now independent in all personal and domestic tasks, managing to socialize once a week and to attend church regularly, and is managing a part-time job (10 hours per week) at her local play school. She hopes in due course to return to her work as a music therapist, but realizes that in order to maintain her health this may be on a part-time basis only.

Case Study 2

Phillip (aged 36) described the onset of his illness as starting shortly after splitting up from his wife 4^1/$_2$ years ago. He stated that this was a particularly stressful time in his life and he noted after the split that he suffered with stomach pains. He went to his GP who diagnosed anxiety and stress. These symptoms eventually went. However, six months later he suffered with 'flu' and was acutely unwell for approximately two weeks. Since this time he has felt generally unwell and described his current symptoms as aches in his arms, neck and head, pain at times, a general lack of energy, nausea, anxiety, low mood and poor sleep.

Phillip described good and bad days, stating that he could do very little on a bad day, apart from wash and dress. On a good day or 'average' day he stated he was able to manage work and occasionally socialize. He stated that he is currently employed in the motor trade, although in general has to have one to three months off intermittently each year. He said that to date his company have been supportive, but he expressed concern about the amount of sick leave he had had to take over the last four years. Phillip lives alone in his own house and stated that although he can work, his domestic chores are generally completed by his mother and his ex-wife. His previous hobbies were going to the gym, playing football and rugby and going to the pub with friends. He said he still occasionally goes to the pub, but suffers for days afterwards.

Phillip has previously tried amitriptyline and Prozac but stated that he could not cope with the side-effects and was currently on no medication. He said he has tried counselling in the past but found it difficult. Phillip's reason for attending the occupational therapy session was for some 'light at the end of the tunnel'.

On attendance at clinic Phillip was placed in the *mild/moderate* level of ability, as although he was still able to attend work his level of ability appeared to fluctuate. He often required time off work. It was agreed at clinic by Phillip, the consultant and the OT as Phillip lived locally the occupational therapy group would be the most appropriate approach to management. Phillip was also interested in meeting other people with the illness as his only previous knowledge was that portrayed in the media, which he often found alarming. The media articles left him believing he did not have CFS as he was not 'bed bound'. Time was spent during the clinic appointment explaining about the different levels of CFS seen, and that not everyone with the illness becomes immobile.

Phillip attended all seven consecutive sessions of the group. During the course of the weeks he was able to try out the techniques discussed and devise his own rest/activity daily plan, which he incorporated into his working day, with the support of his boss.

Phillip particularly found the relaxation techniques extremely effective, using a variety of autogenic methods, breathing exercises and resting positions during his rest periods. By talking to others in the group of a similar activity level to his own, Phillip became very motivated to attempt the techniques and change a number of aspects within his lifestyle. In particular, he levelled out the peaks and troughs so that he no longer had 'good' and 'bad' days. He divided up the activities he wanted to achieve into smaller components and said 'no' to social events such as going to the pub if he had exceeded his high-energy load for that day or week.

On attendance at the follow-up session (three months after attendance at the group) Phillip said he had experienced up and downs and had had to make frequent changes to his timetable but that overall he had an increased activity level and was no longer peaking and troughing.

At the one-year follow-up clinic appointment Phillip had sustained his improvement in activity levels, was able to manage work without frequent sickness absence and was managing his own shopping but his mother still assisted with laundry and vacuuming. He commented that he could probably do these chores for himself but that his mother seemed to like to do them! Phillip added that he had also restarted counselling to assist with his understanding of why his relationship with his wife had not worked. Phillip had stayed in touch with the CFS team and rang for advice as required. This was generally every couple of months.

Case Study 3

Fiona (aged 48) described her illness as starting six years ago following a 'flu-like' illness from which she felt she never recovered. She described her current symptoms on attendance at the occupational therapy initial session as extreme tiredness, daily headache, general weakness, aching neck, sensitivity to light and tinnitus. She stated that at the onset of the illness she had been unable to keep her balance. At times she had collapsed and been taken to her local hospital for investigations but no cause for her symptoms had been identified.

Fiona stated that she lived with her husband and two children aged 14 and 16 in their own house. She said she could manage her own self-care but needed her husband's assistance with domestic chores, especially the shopping. She could walk indoors but needed a wheelchair outdoors. At the onset of the illness Fiona was a librarian; she had not worked since the onset. Fiona stated that she had experienced a number of stressful events in the last 10 years, these being a car crash, a number of bereavements, moving house and undergoing a hysterectomy nine years ago.

She said she had recently been started on 20 mg of amitriptyline two hours prior to bed at night, and although this assisted her with getting off to sleep, she was still waking frequently during the night. On waking in the morning she did not feel refreshed.

She said she had previously enjoyed gardening and attempted to do gentle exercises at home, but often overdid it and would need to rest for a number of days before attempting to recommence her exercise routine. Her reason for attendance at the occupational therapy session was to learn as much as possible.

At clinic Fiona's level of ability was defined as *moderate/severe*. During the course of Fiona's clinic appointment the possibility of an inpatient admission was discussed owing to her level of ability and the distance she lived from the unit. However, Fiona stated she would prefer to attempt management as an outpatient initially and a two-hour occupational therapy session was agreed.

On attendance at the session with her husband, Fiona described her purpose for attending as:

(1) To learn as much as possible.

During the session Fiona was introduced to the concepts of:

- the pattern of peaks and troughs that can affect daily life;
- the importance of having a structured day, and balancing rest and activity throughout the day. An individual rest and activity plan was

devised for Fiona which incorporated four half-hour rest period spaced evenly throughout her day;
- what is meant by rest and activity and the use of relaxation techniques to enable effective rest;
- the need to establish a baseline of activity, and to consider energy requirements and the importance of pacing activity;
- the need to reintroduce activity in a gradual and systematic way over time, with the use of goal planning and breaking activities down into achievable chunks;
- the importance of having realistic and achievable goals in order to achieve personal aims;
- the influence on the illness of feelings and thoughts and ways of identifying, challenging and changing any recurring negative thought patterns;
- the effect of the illness on friends and family relationships.

During the course of the session Fiona identified that she was currently pushing herself to achieve an unrealistic amount of activity for her level of current ability. She was able to see the importance of achieving a consistent baseline and was encouraged to keep a diary to assist in identifying her baseline. Fiona was encouraged to work on her aims in a more gradual and systematic way by steadily increasing her activity over time.

Fiona was given contact details for the OT and encouraged to make contact for ongoing advice and support. Fiona did contact the team four months following her initial session for a further face-to-face follow-up session. Her main reason for requesting the session was that she was finding it extremely difficult to 'stick to the timetable'.

On discussion at the follow-up session it was obvious that Fiona had made some changes to her lifestyle. She no longer pushed herself but had not being able to establish a daily rest/activity plan and tended to do most of her activity in the morning and rest all afternoon. The importance of a balanced day was reinforced and discussed in depth during the session. It was also apparent during the session that Fiona was finding it difficult to come to terms with her diagnosis and stated that she wanted a 'magic solution' to her difficulties. She said that although she understood the principles of the education into the management of CFS, doing it 'day in, day out' was very difficult.

It was agreed that Fiona needed more time to discuss the management principles and to come to terms with her illness, and she was encouraged to reconsider coming into hospital for the inpatient programme. Her husband supported this idea; however, Fiona said she would try again at home. Regular contact with the OT was encouraged.

Over the following two years, Fiona made steady progress with weekly, then two-weekly and then monthly contact with the OT to review her goals and daily rest/activity plan. She is now mobile without her wheelchair indoors and outdoors, can manage most domestic chores although the family carries these out on a rota basis and she has recommenced gardening. Fiona was keen to start an exercise programme and was encouraged to slowly introduce walking; she can now manage a half-hour walk daily and aims to increase this over time so that she can walk into the town, three miles away.

Case Study 4

Michael (aged 25), on inpatient admission to the CFS Service, was unable to tolerate any sound or light and required assistance in all areas of daily life. He had been predominantly in bed at home for two years prior to admission, only able to transfer to the wheelchair to go to the toilet two to three times a day. His mother had given up her job as a secretary to care for Michael full time. Conversation was limited to short five- to 10-minute sessions two to three times a day. Michael described a disturbed sleep pattern, at times sleeping during the day and being awake at night, or continuously catnapping, with no deep or extended sleep. On observation Michael was extremely thin as he found it difficult to eat enough to sustain his weight because of the energy required to chew and to swallow.

Over a period of time it was possible to gain a history of the illness from Michael and his parents. The illness had started four years previously when Michael was in his final year of university. Michael did not recall a specific illness at the outset. However, he described feeling increasingly tired throughout his third year at university and eventually had to return home. He was unable to return to university to complete his studies. He had attempted to restart activity prior to admission but said he never seemed to get beyond a certain point and always relapsed after some weeks. He stated that it would then take weeks or months to regain his previous level (which was never more than being able to transfer and wash and feed himself).

Prior to admission Michael's illness dominated the house; in an attempt to limit noise his mother no longer used the vacuum cleaner or mowed the lawn, and the curtains in the house were permanently drawn to restrict light.

On admission to hospital Michael needed some weeks to adjust to being in hospital. His level of ability was defined as *very severe*. The initial goals were based around desensitizing Michael to light and sound by opening his curtains for short periods during the day. He was encouraged to sit out in a chair, initially for two minutes once a day building to 10 minutes three times a day. This was based on Michael's aim of sitting out in a chair for his meals, and ultimately feeding himself.

Michael's initial aims were:

(1) To feed himself.
(2) To wash and dress himself.
(3) To go out to the toilet in a wheelchair rather than using the commode or bedpan.

Over the following 12 weeks as an inpatient Michael achieved the above aims but this used all his energy.

His next aim was to start to have some cognitive stimulation again, in particular to be able to read and write, watch television and use a computer. In addition he wanted to walk and climb stairs. Each of these aims was broken down into small components and slowly introduced into Michael's day.

During the establishment of these aims, Michael found he was becoming more and more emotional and asked to return home for a recess. Contact was made with a local psychologist who had previously been involved in Michael's management, to address the emotional issues that were currently limiting Michael's activity level. Michael stated that his emotional level has a lot to do with a fear of the unknown, and the possibility of relapse.

Michael returned home for six months, where he continued to work on his goals; he then returned to the unit for a short top-up admission of three weeks, to adapt his timetable and the goal plan.

Since his initial admission four years ago Michael has stayed in regular contact with the team. He is now independent in all activities of daily living, has managed to go on two holidays and has just started at his local university part time to complete his degree in electronics. However, it is not a straightforward progression up the ladder, and he has on many occasions had to re-establish his baseline, because he has contracted a cold, or at times overdone it. He has used each episode as part of the learning process and always contacted the team for support and guidance as required, initially by letter and later, as his speech and ability to sustain a conversation improved, by telephone.

Section Five:
Research, Measurement
and Future Directions

There are a number of different aspects of chronic fatigue syndrome (CFS) that would need to be considered to examine the effect of treatment programmes for research and clinical evaluation. The Royal Colleges (1996) and the National Task Force (1994) concurred that a multidisciplinary approach, with expert assessment for more complex cases, and a goal-orientated programme are required for management of patients with CFS. Research studies are needed to assess each of these components and to identify which aspects are required for which patients.

In addition, it is unclear from previous studies whether the appropriate setting for treatment and management is primary care (community), secondary care (outpatient) or tertiary care (inpatient), and whether this is dependent on specific patient characteristics.

Studies often require recruitment over an extended period owing to the relatively small number of patients with CFS seen in local units. Future studies will need to take this into account to ensure adequate statistical power throughout the studies to detect treatment effect. A possible solution to the recruitment issues would be the establishment of a multicentre trial. In this instance, the therapy would need to be clearly defined as a 'black box' of therapy, as the cognitive behaviour therapy and/or occupational therapy programme carried out at one centre may not be the same as at other centres (Pemberton et al., 1994; Sharpe et al., 1996; Deale et al., 1997; Essame et al., 1998; Cox, 1999a).

Chapter 10 will discuss aspects of measurement and suggest a number of selected scales for use in the clinical and research settings. Chapter 11 will then discuss the type of possible approaches that could be utilized to structure services and aid patient management.

Chapter 10
Measurement

A number of different aspects have been identified by the author that would need to be considered in evaluating a person with chronic fatigue syndrome (CFS), namely:

- functional status;
- perceived general health;
- fatigue;
- disability;
- coping;
- somatic signs;
- mood and psychological disorder.

Each of these components will now be considered. Scales of measurement have been identified by the author that have either been used in other studies (see Table 5.1) and/or have being designed specifically for CFS. These are given in Table 10.1. The list is not exhaustive and should be viewed as possible suggestions for assessment of occupational therapy interventions for clinical evaluation and research.

Functional Status and Perceived Health

Occupational Therapy Lifestyle Management for CFS (see Chapter 9) aims to teach strategies to change behaviour, attitudes and beliefs and accordingly promote a change in the level of activity (Cox, 1998, 1999a). Functional status and change in activity levels are therefore important outcomes of an occupational therapy programme. Scales have been considered which measure these constructs.

A number of activity of daily living scales were reviewed (Jette, 1985; Eakin, 1989a, 1989b; Bowling, 1991, 1995; Jeffery, 1993), such as the Barthel Index (Mahoney and Barthel, 1965). It was felt that this type of scale would be difficult to use owing to a lack of sensitivity to functional status in CFS.

Table 10.1: Selected measurement scales for CFS

Name of scale	SF-36	Health and Fatigue Questionnaire	Profile of Fatigue Related Symptoms (PFRS)	Social Adjustment Questionnaire	Illness Management Questionnaire (IMQ)	Hospital Anxiety and Depression Scale (HAD)
Authors	Stewart et al., 1988 Ware et al., 1993	Chalder et al., 1993 Pawlikowska et al., 1994	Ray et al., 1992a	Chalder et al., 1996	Ray et al., 1993	Zigmond and Snaith, 1983
Designed to assess	To survey differences in physical and mental health status, and the effect of treatment on general health status	To measure severity of fatigue, detection of fatigue, and as a valid estimator of change in hospital and community settings	To assess patient's severity and pattern of CFS, and evaluate the effects of treatment	To assess disability and functional impairment	To assess coping in CFS, and to provide a measure of coping which is problem focused rather than directed toward the management of distress	To aid the clinician to assess anxiety and depression
Type of scale	Self-administered Likert-type scale for persons 14 years or older	Self-rating adjectival scale	Self-rating multidimensional measure 54 items asked about the past week	Self-administered visual analogue scale	Self-rated numerical response scale	Self-administered Likert-type scale
Subscales	Physical functioning Social functioning	Physical fatigue Mental fatigue Length of current tiredness	Emotional distress Cognitive difficulty	Ability to work Home management	Maintaining activity	Anxiety Depression

Role functioning: physical Body pain Mental health Role functioning: emotional Vitality General health	Percentage of time tired	Fatigue Somatic symptoms	Social leisure Private leisure Relationships	Accommodating to illness Focusing on symptoms Information seeking	4-point scale which relates to a numerical score from 0 to 3 The higher the score the worse the anxiety and/or depression. A score of less than 8 is considered non-pathological
Scoring — Raw scores are transformed into a 0 to 100 scale (percentage value)	Bimodal response system (0, 0, 1, 1) or Likert scoring (0, 1, 2, 3)	7-point scale, raw scores used to compute means	9-point scale, with the highest score representing the greatest degree of difficulty	6-point scale, the score for each subscale is computed by summing the scores on the items belonging to each scale, and dividing by the number of items	
Validity and reliability — Good construct validity, internal consistency, test-retest reliability and sensitive to change (Brazier et al., 1992)	Good face validity, high levels of internal reliability and sensitive to change	High estimates for convergent validity, test-retest reliability and internal consistency	Unclear, however has been used in a number of CFS trials (Butler et al., 1991; Bonner et al., 1994; Deale et al., 1997)	Reliability and validity unclear, however the scale correlates highly with other scales	Reliable guide to the type of mood disorder which is biological in origin such as a depressed state most likely to respond to antidepressants

(contd)

Table 10.1: (contd)

Name of scale	SF-36	Health and Fatigue Questionnaire	Profile of Fatigue Related Symptoms (PFRS)	Social Adjustment Questionnaire	Illness Management Questionnaire (IMQ)	Hospital Anxiety and Depression Scale (HAD)
General comments	In the clinical setting it needs to be administered before the respondent sees the provider to limit influence in the respondent's answers	Designed specifically with fatigue in mind. Easy to score and interpret	Designed specifically for CFS. Differentiates between components of fatigue within CFS	Easy to administer and score. Quick indication of level of impairment	Specifically designed for CFS. Gives detailed information on range of coping. Takes time to interpret scores. Better as research tool	Quick and easily interpreted

The Sickness Impact Profile was considered, as it was designed as a measure of perceived health status (Bergner et al., 1981), that is, how the patient perceives the impact of illness or trauma on his/her life. The Sickness Impact Profile concentrates on assessing the impact of sickness on daily activities and behaviour, rather than feelings and clinical reports. The profile takes 20–30 minutes. It is felt that the CFS patient group may not be able to complete such a lengthy scale in addition to other measures.

The Short Form Health Survey Questionnaire (SF-36) (Stewart et al., 1988; Ware et al., 1993) appears to be worth consideration. The SF-36 was constructed to survey differences in physical and mental health status, the health burden of chronic disease and other medical conditions, and the effect of treatments on general health status. It was designed for use in clinical practice, research, health policy evaluations and general population surveys (Ware and Sherbourne, 1992). The UK version has slight modifications to make it more appropriate for UK populations (Brazier et al., 1992).

In addition, although no specific functional scales for CFS were identified, the inclusion of a global measure of functional improvement may assist in evaluating the overall impact of a treatment programme on individuals. Other studies with CFS patients have used the Karnofsky scale (Karnofsky et al., 1948) as a crude measure of functional change to good effect (Sharpe et al., 1996; Essame et al., 1998).

Fatigue

No universal definition of fatigue exists but the nervous system is postulated to play a significant role in the perception and modulation of fatigue (Piper, 1997). Fatigue in CFS is now considered to be subjective and central in origin (Wessely and Thomas, 1990), and is a multidimensional construct that can be positively or negatively influenced by activity, exercises, rest, sleep, disease, symptoms and psychological patterns (Piper, 1997). Although fatigue is non-specific and highly subjective it is a predominant complaint in many disorders (Krupp et al., 1989).

A number of scales that assess fatigue were evaluated (Krupp et al., 1989; Schwartz et al., 1993; Fisk et al., 1994) but because of the subjective nature of fatigue, scales that had been designed specifically for CFS were felt to be more sensitive.

Fatigue is the most prevalent symptom of CFS, yet the natural history of fatigue and its reliable and valid measurement remain relatively undeveloped (Barofsky and Legro, 1991). Owing to its subjective nature, fatigue has proved difficult to define (David et al., 1988; Sharpe et al., 1991) and its features may vary dependent upon the illness content (Barofsky and Legro, 1991).

Two specific scales designed for the CFS population were identified: (1) the Health and Fatigue Questionnaire (Chalder et al., 1993); (2) the Profile of Fatigue Related Symptoms (PFRS; Ray et al., 1992a). Both scales attempt to define and reflect the dimension of fatigue. Chalder and colleagues (1993) identified the fact that many synonyms are used to describe fatigue, and worded differently it means different things to different people. Words used such as exhaustion, general fatigue, feeling tired all the time or feeling weak could all mean fatigue. The many synonyms used are therefore reflected in the scale. They conclude that fatigue is viewed better as a dimension rather than a category. A distinction is made between mental and physical fatigue, as this is specific to CFS.

The term fatigue was not used in the PFRS for the same reason as in the Health and Fatigue Questionnaire, that is, it means different things to different people. During the development of the PFRS, a distinction emerged between fatigue and cognitive difficulty, as noted previously by Wessely and Powell (1989). However, rather than defining this as mental and physical fatigue (Chalder et al., 1993), Ray and colleagues (1992a) used the term cognitive difficulty to emphasize the distinct nature of the factor. The PFRS highlights symptoms most closely identified with CFS.

Disability

One aspect of assessing functional status is to see how this impacts on a individual's life, and through this assessment to evaluate the level of disability. The Social Adjustment Questionnaire, as used by Chalder and colleagues (1996), has been designed specifically for the CFS population to assess disability. It was constructed as a self-assessment scale of functional impairment and as a measure of disability.

Specific Symptoms

As described in Chapter, 1, CFS is a multidimensional syndrome of many symptoms, not just fatigue. Scales that measured these other symptoms were considered for their specificity to CFS. Somatic symptoms are assessed in the PFRS scale, which has been specifically designed for a CFS population. In addition, the somatic scale of the PFRS was found to have a high correlation with the Modified Somatic Perception Questionnaire (Main, 1983) and with the somatization dimension of the Brief Symptom Inventory (Ray et al., 1992a).

The PFRS also considered emotional distress and cognitive difficulties (Ray et al., 1992a). When developing the PFRS (1992a) found that little research had been done on the structure of symptoms within the illness, nor had explicit consideration been given to how symptoms should be assessed. They concluded that appropriate and easily administered measures were required to assess patients in terms of both the severity and pattern of their illness, and to monitor the effects of treatment (Ray et al., 1992a). Of the many scales previously used in CFS research, the majority had not been developed with the range of symptoms associated with CFS in mind. In a recent study Ray and colleagues (1997) found that poorer outcomes in CFS were predicted by subjective cognitive difficulty and somatic symptoms, and that anxiety, depression and emotional distress appeared to have no influence.

Coping

Style of coping and illness management are major components in assessing treatment effect as cognitive behaviour therapy (CBT) examines patients' beliefs and attitudes about illness and pinpoints ways to manage and overcome illness, by identifying how the illness affects thoughts, feelings and behaviour (Sharpe, 1991; Cox and Findley, 1998; Cox, 1998).

The way people cope with stress has been studied in various forms over the years (Carver et al., 1989; Blakeley et al., 1991; Epstein and Katz, 1992). Carver and colleagues (1989) divided coping into active coping (the process of taking active steps to try to remove or circumvent a stressor or ameliorate its effects) and planning (thinking how to cope with a stressor). Ray and colleagues (1992b) expanded on this concept and developed the Illness Management Questionnaire to assess illness-focused coping in CFS, and it is composed of items directly pertinent to the disorder.

The Illness Management Questionnaire was designed (Ray et al., 1993) to assess coping in CFS and to provide a measure of coping which is problem focused rather than directed toward the management of distress. It has been suggested that the Illness Management Questionnaire may be employed to relate ways of coping to outcomes in CFS, and to assess coping as a mediator of change in cognitive-behavioural interventions. In a recent study (Ray et al., 1997) the level of fatigue experienced was predicated on information seeking and impairment on behavioural disengagement and a low internal locus of control. The belief that action can influence outcome modified the relationship between illness accommodation and both fatigue and impairment.

Mood and Psychological Disorder

CFS has been strongly associated with depression (Wessely and Powell, 1989). Previous studies have identified that 50–80% of patients with CFS also meet the criteria for the diagnosis of major depression (Hickie et al., 1995). Both CFS and major depression list fatigue, sleep disturbance, psychomotor changes, cognitive impairment and mood changes as characteristic features (Lloyd et al., 1990a).

However, most CFS patients rarely report weight loss, guilt or suicidal ideation, and do not have observable psychomotor slowing (Hickie et al., 1995). Patients with CFS tend to be irritable and have transient depression rather than a profound loss of interest in daily activities. Some 25% of CFS patients also fulfil the criteria for anxiety and somatization disorder (Wessely, 1992; Hickie et al., 1995).

Wessely and Thomas (1990) suggested that at least half of the CFS patients seen in a general hospital will have a disorder of mood, and that the management of affective disorder is an essential part of the treatment of CFS. Ray and colleagues (1992b) concluded that fatigue, somatic symptoms and cognitive difficulty were associated with general illness severity but emotional distress was not, thus negative emotions did not contribute directly to patients' perception of illness severity. They argue that the correlation reflects a reciprocal influence, with negative emotions exacerbating fatigue and other symptoms and the debilitating nature of their symptoms enhancing emotional vulnerability.

In a recent review, Sharpe and colleagues (1997) asserted that anxiety disorder may be more common in patients who present with fatigue than previously realized. Suicide is the only recognized cause of death in CFS (Wessely and Thomas, 1990; Sharpe et al., 1997). Therefore, examination of mood is required in the assessment of CFS. Patients with CFS who are still ill have been shown to have significantly higher depression and anxiety scores on the Hospital Anxiety and Depression Scale than those who are well (Wood et al., 1992), although the mean scores were generally at a non-pathological level. Patients still suffering from CFS therefore had significantly more emotional distress than those that had recovered (Wood et al., 1992). However, it has been shown that the psychological disturbance experienced is likely to be a consequence of the illness rather than an antecedent risk factor of the syndrome (Hickie et al., 1990).

Mood is also reflected in the SF-36 Mental Health concept which assesses depression, anxiety, behavioural emotional control and general positive affect, and the Emotional Role Functioning concept which assesses the extent to which emotional problems interfere with work or other daily activities, such as decreased time and accomplishing less. In addition, the PFRS Emotional Distress subscale assesses depression, anxiety and anger, defined as a single factor.

Conclusion

Goal setting is a major component of the Occupational Therapy Lifestyle Management programme and of CBT (Surawy et al., 1995; Cox and Findley, 1998, see Chapter 9). In research studies an evaluation of goals set prior to discharge could be utilized as a better indicator of improvement in ability than symptom reduction and general health.

Overall, a variety of measures would be required owing to the complexity and variability of CFS. Such measures might be the PFRS, Illness Management Questionnaire, Health and Fatigue Questionnaire and the Karnofsky scale and goal achievement evaluation.

Chapter 11
Future Directions

The occupational therapy chronic fatigue syndrome (CFS) intervention discussed involves further input following discharge from the admission, group or consultation than just the sessions alone, to ensure change in lifestyle and therefore enable change in the patient's activity level, as the case studies aimed to illustrate. This has implications for practice, and the study by Essame and colleagues (1998) supports this observation. They noted that, following inpatient treatment:

> ...outpatient progress was more easily maintained if a good working relationship was developed between the team and carer [and that] adequate and appropriate follow-up was important for continued improvement. (p.56)

A recent report (National Task Force, 1998) highlighted the need for primary care, outpatient treatment and inpatient care for patients unable to cope with outpatient management. However, the report also states that CFS services are limited. As a consequence of the limited services in the UK the service described has a national catchment area. Follow up from the service is therefore dependent on the patient contacting his/her occupational therapist (OT) at the hospital for further adaptation and modification of the individual programme by letter or telephone, and/or on the support of local OTs to continue with the same approach at home (Cox, 1998, 1999a). On occasions, inpatients were readmitted six months to one year after their original admission to adapt their programme and reassess their level of functioning (Cox, 1998). It has been suggested that problems with management can arise if primary care teams do not share the same approach (Essame et al., 1998).

There are a number of models of care that may be useful to consider to guide this follow-up contact, in particular, shared care (Edwards et al., 1996), case management (Holloway et al., 1995), care management (Russell-Hodgson, 1998) and home care (Hughes et al., 1997).

Edwards and colleagues (1996) describe shared care as:

...primary and secondary care clinicians having joint care for the patient [which means] ...in essence the general practitioner (GP) remains centrally involved in the care of patients who have been referred to specialists. (p. xii)

Shared care requires the establishment of standards of care that are agreed by all those involved (Edwards et al., 1996). In order for shared care to work effectively, training of the primary care teams in the approach used at the centre would be required (National Task Force, 1998), as the model involves the active participation of the GP and primary care team in the management of their patient with CFS prior to, during and following an admission or outpatient treatment.

Case management was considered, as it has been used in the management of psychiatric patients who would have long-term contact needs similar to those of the patient with CFS (Holloway et al., 1995). Case management involves one person acting as a key worker and following the patient throughout his/her care pathway (Holloway et al., 1995). This is a similar model to the management approach already used within the team, in that the OT acts as a key worker for further advice and guidance following discharge (Cox, 1998, 1999a). The disadvantage with this model for the CFS service is that it depends on formal booked contact times. The Occupational Therapy Lifestyle Management programme places the responsibility of contacting the service with the patient when required, not with the therapist (Cox and Findley, 1998; Cox, 1999a), thus relying on a collaborative rather than led approach (Sharpe et al., 1997). Formal booked contact times may also not be an effective use of time for either patient or therapist, as it may be more appropriate to have contact when there are issues that the patient wishes to discuss. In addition, currently there is no one model of case management, and the different models need to be compared (Holloway et al., 1995).

Care management involves collaborative joint working between the health and social care sectors (Russell-Hodgson, 1998). The system was developed to assess care needs and arrange services to meet those needs under the legislative framework of the National Health Service and Community Care Act, 1990 (Tanner, 1998). The model utilizes a key-worker approach that is often client led. Personnel, usually from the local social services department, are placed within a health care facility. The aim is to aid communication and accessibility, and therefore bridge the gap between the two service providers: health, and social services (Russell-Hodgson, 1998). This approach may be useful with patients who have a high need for social care interventions such as equipment, adaptations and social care packages. However, the majority of patients with CFS would not need this level of collaboration with social services and therefore this may not be a useful model to consider.

Home care is defined as the delivery of nursing, medical, or support services in patients' homes (Hughes et al., 1997). Although home care has been shown to be beneficial in reducing acute hospital days for terminally ill or elderly patients (Hughes et al., 1997), it was not felt to be an appropriate model of care for the CFS population. The main reasons for rejecting this model centre on the fact that it would involve the OTs in a considerable amount of travelling because of the national catchment area of this centre, and that the programme is based philosophically on rehabilitation rather than care (Cox, 1999a). However, this may be an appropriate model for a primary-care-based team to consider.

Shared care would therefore appear to be the more appropriate model to consider. Although the results in the management of asthma and diabetes have been ambiguous, overall studies have indicated that shared care can be as effective as hospital care (Greenhalgh, 1994; Eastwood and Sheldon, 1996). The Royal Colleges (1996) emphasized that most patients with CFS should be managed in primary care, and that there are a number of patients who will require more specialist inpatient care. With appropriate training the shared care model may therefore be the interface between the two extremes of care currently available (Edwards et al., 1996; National Task Force, 1998).

OTs are based in all areas of the health and social care sectors (Paterson, 1998), so are well placed to assist in the transition from hospital to primary care. In addition, OTs are trained in addressing the problems of motivation in patients who have a long path to recovery (Mattingly, 1994). One of the main difficulties often encountered in CFS management is the lack of sustained improvement in physical changes when regular contact for further advice and management is not available (Cox, 1999b). If more regular local contact were available with an OT based in the primary care setting and trained in the approach, this observation might be different.

In the interim period prior to the necessary education of primary care teams being completed, integrated care pathways may be a solution to aid the management of CFS (Rossiter et al., 1998). Integrated care pathways utilize continuous documentation that details the expected intervention and incorporates long- and short-term goals. They have been shown to be valuable in the monitoring of the rehabilitation process and in demonstrating effectiveness in terms of goal achievement in multiple sclerosis (Rossiter et al., 1998).

A major emphasis of the programme is to diagnose and evaluate patients appropriately under one roof rather than attending hospital for numerous outpatient visits. The aim is to contain the cost to the patient in terms of fatigue and finance. In addition, many of the inpatients admitted to the programme leave with an alternative diagnosis (Cox and Findley, 1998). This highlights the importance of a multi-skilled team to complete the assessment and management process using a biopsychosocial approach (Royal Colleges, 1996).

It has been suggested that rather than being from a specific professional discipline the clinician or therapist should be in possession of the appropriate knowledge, skills and attitudes for the most effective management of CFS (Wessely et al., 1998). The OTs in the centre described have gained this knowledge, skill and attitude base over a number of years, and have completed additional training in cognitive behaviour therapy (CBT) (Cox, 1998, 1999a). In 1998, Sharpe stated that:

> ...treatment with CBT requires a skilled therapist – and few such therapists are available. (p. 61)

Training of the multi-professional team will therefore be essential in the management of CFS (Royal Colleges, 1996; National Task Force, 1998).

References

Acheson S (1959) The clinical syndrome variously called benign myalgic encephalomyelitis, Iceland disease and epidemic neuromyasthenia (first published in American Journal of Medicine: 569–95). In The Clinical and Scientific Basis of Myalgic Encephalomyelitis/Chronic Fatigue Syndrome. Ottawa: Nightingale Research Foundation (1992), pp. 129–58.

Andrews G (1996) Talk that works: the rise of cognitive behaviour therapy. British Medical Journal 313: 1501–2.

Armon C, Kurland LT (1991) Chronic fatigue syndrome: issues in the diagnosis and estimation of incidence. Reviews of Infectious Diseases 13(Suppl 1): S68–72.

Barofsky I, Legro MW (1991) Definition and measurement of fatigue. Reviews of Infectious Diseases 13(Suppl 1): S94–7.

Bates DW, Schmitt W, Buchwald D, Ware NC, Lee J, Thoyer E, Kornish J, Komaroff AL (1993) Prevalence of fatigue and chronic fatigue syndrome in a primary care practice. Archives of Internal Medicine 152: 2759–65.

Bates DW, Buchwald D, Lee J, Kith P, Doolittle T, Rutherford C, Churchill WH, Schur PH, Werner M, Wybenga D, Winkleman J, Komaroff AL (1995) Clinical laboratory test findings in patients with chronic fatigue syndrome. Archives of Internal Medicine 155: 97–103.

Bearn J, Wessely S (1994) Neurobiological aspects of the chronic fatigue syndrome. European Journal of Clinical Investigation 24: 79–90.

Beck AT (1976) Cognitive Therapy and the Emotional Disorders. New York: International United Press.

Behan PO, Behan WMH (1988) Postviral Fatigue Syndrome. CRC Critical Reviews in Neurobiology 4(2): 157–78.

Behan PO, Hanniffah BAG, Doogan DO, Loudon M (1994) A pilot study of sertraline for the treatment of chronic fatigue syndrome. Journal of Clinical Infectious Diseases 18(Suppl): S111.

Behan WMH, More IAR, Behan PO (1991) Mitochondrial abnormalities in the postviral fatigue syndrome. Acta Neuropathologica 83: 61–5.

Bell D (1992) Chronic fatigue syndrome. Recent advances in diagnosis and treatment. Postgraduate Medicine 91(6): 245–52.

Bennett RM (1989) Physical fitness and muscle metabolism in the fibromyalgia syndrome: an overview. Journal of Rheumatology S19(16): 28–9.

Bergner M, Bobbitt RA, Carter WB, Gilson BS (1981) The Sickness Impact Profile: development and final revision of a health status measure. Medical Care 19(8): 787–805.

Blakeley AA, Howard RC, Sosich RM, Murdoch JC, Menkes DB, Spears GS (1991) Psychiatric symptoms, personality and ways of coping in chronic fatigue syndrome. Psychological Medicine 21: 347–62.

Bonner D, Ron M, Chalder T, Butler S, Wessely S (1994) Chronic fatigue syndrome: a follow up study. Journal of Neurology, Neurosurgery and Psychiatry 57: 617–21.

Bou-Holaigah I, Rowe PC, Kan J, Calkins H (1995) The relationship between neurally mediated hypotension and the chronic fatigue syndrome. Journal of the American Medical Association 274(12): 961–7.

Bowling A (1991) Measuring Health: A Review of Quality of Life Measurement Scales. Milton Keynes: Open University Press.

Bowling A (1995) Measuring Disease: A Review of Disease-specific Quality of Life Measurement Scales. Milton Keynes: Open University Press.

Brazier JE, Harper R, Jones NMB, O'Cathain A, Thomas KJ, Usherwood T, Westlake L (1992) Validating the SF-36 health survey questionnaire: new outcome measure for primary care. British Medical Journal 305(6846): 160–4.

Bryder L (1987) Occupational therapy and tuberculosis. Society for Social History of Medicine Bulletin 40: 64–6.

Buchwald D, Komaroff AL (1991) Review of laboratory findings for patients with chronic fatigue syndrome. Reviews of Infectious Diseases 13(Suppl 1): S12–18.

Buchwald D, Garrity D (1994) Comparison of patients with chronic fatigue syndrome, fibromyalgia, and multiple chemical sensitivities. Archives of Internal Medicine 154: 2049-53.

Buchwald D, Sullivan JL, Komaroff AL (1987) Frequency of 'chronic active Epstein–Barr virus infection' in a general medical practice. Journal of the American Medical Association 257: 2303–7.

Buchwald D, Pearlman T, Kith P, Katon W, Schmaling K (1997) Screening for psychiatric disorders in chronic fatigue and chronic fatigue syndrome. Journal of Psychosomatic Research 42(1): 87–94.

Buchwald D, Umali P, Umali J, Kith P, Pearlman T, Komaroff AL (1995) Chronic fatigue and the chronic fatigue syndrome: prevalence in a Pacific Northwest health care system. Annals of Internal Medicine 123: 81–8.

Butler S, Chalder T, Ron M, Wessely S (1991) Cognitive behaviour therapy in chronic fatigue syndrome. Journal of Neurology, Neurosurgery and Psychiatry 54: 153–8.

Calder BD, Warnock PJ, McCartney RA, Bell EJ (1987) Coxsackie B viruses and the postviral syndrome: a prospective study in general practice. Journal of the Royal College of General Practitioners 37: 11–14.

Canadian Association of Occupational Therapists (CAOT) (1991) Occupational Therapy Guidelines for Client Centred Practice. Toronto: Canadian Association of Occupational Therapists.

Carver CS, Scheier MF, Wientraub JK (1989) Assessing coping strategies: a theoretically based approach. Journal of Personality and Social Psychology 56(2): 267–83.

Chalder T (1997) Cognitive-behavioural treatment approach for patients with CFS. British Journal of Therapy and Rehabilitation 4(12): 655–8.

Chalder T, Berelowitz G, Pawlikowska T, Watts L, Wessely S, Wright D, Wallace EP (1993) Development of a fatigue scale. Journal of Psychosomatic Research 37(2): 147–53.

Chalder T, Deale A, Wessely S, Marks I (1995) Cognitive behaviour therapy for chronic fatigue syndrome (letter). American Journal of Medicine 98: 419–20.

Chalder T, Butler S, Wessely S (1996) Inpatient treatment of chronic fatigue syndrome. Behavioural and Cognitive Psychotherapy 24: 351–65.

Chalder T, Power MJ, Wessely S (1996) Chronic fatigue in the community: 'A question of attribution'. Psychological Medicine 26: 791–800.

Chevalier M (1997) Occupational therapy and the search for meaning. British Journal of Occupational Therapy 60(12): 539–40.

Christiansen C, Baum C (1997a) Understanding occupation: definitions and concepts. In Christiansen C, Baum C (Eds) Occupational Therapy: Enabling Function and Well Being, 2nd edn. New Jersey: Slack, Ch. 1.

Christiansen C, Baum C (1997b) Person–environment occupational performance: a conceptual model for practice. In Christiansen C, Baum C (Eds) Occupational Therapy: Enabling Function and Well Being, 2nd edn. New Jersey: Slack, Ch. 3.

Christodoulou C, DeLuca J, Lange G, Johnson SK, Sisto SA, Korn L, Natelson BH (1998) Relation between neuropsychological impairment and functional disability in patients with chronic fatigue syndrome. Journal of Neurology, Neurosurgery and Psychiatry 64: 431–4.

Clark MR, Katon W, Russo J, Kith P, Sintay M, Buchwald D (1995) Chronic fatigue: risk factors for symptom persistence in a $2^1/_2$ year follow up study. American Journal of Medicine 98: 187–95.

Cleare AJ (1997) Psychiatric aspects of chronic fatigue syndrome. British Journal of Therapy and Rehabilitation 4(12): 659–62.

Cleare AJ, Bearn J, Allain T, McGregor A, Wessely S, Murray RM, O'Keane V (1995) Contrasting neuroendocrine responses in depression and chronic fatigue syndrome. Journal of Affective Disorders 35: 283–9.

Clements A, Sharpe M, Simkin S, Borrill J, Hawton K (1997) Chronic fatigue syndrome: a qualitative investigation of patients' beliefs about the illness. Journal of Psychosomatic Research 42(6): 615–24.

College of Occupational Therapists (1994) Core Skills and a Conceptual Foundation for Practice: A Position Statement. London: College of Occupational Therapists.

Compston ND (1978) An outbreak of encephalomyelitis in the Royal Free Hospital Group, London, in 1955. Postgraduate Medical Journal 54: 722–4.

Cope H, David AS (1996) Neuroimaging in chronic fatigue syndrome. Journal of Neurology, Neurosurgery and Psychiatry 60: 471–3.

Cope H, David A, Pelosi A, Mann A (1994) Predictors of chronic 'postviral' fatigue. Lancet 344: 864–8.

Cox DL (1998) Management of CFS: development and evaluation of a service. British Journal of Therapy and Rehabilitation 5(4): 205–9.

Cox DL (1999a) Chronic fatigue syndrome: an occupational therapy programme. Occupational Therapy International 6(1): 52–64.

Cox DL (1999b) An evaluation of an occupational therapy in-patient intervention for chronic fatigue syndrome. PhD Thesis, King's College, London.

Cox DL, Findley LJ (1994) Is chronic fatigue syndrome treatable in an NHS environment? Clinical Rehabilitation 8(1): 76–80.

Cox DL, Findley LJ (1998) The management of chronic fatigue syndrome in an inpatient setting: presentation of an approach and perceived outcome. British Journal of Occupational Therapy 61(9): 405–9.

Cox IM, Campbell MJ, Dowson D (1991) Red blood cell magnesium and chronic fatigue syndrome. Lancet 337: 757–60.

Creek (1997a) The knowledge base of occupational therapy. In Creek J (Ed) Occupational Therapy and Mental Health, 2nd edn. Edinburgh: Churchill Livingstone, Ch. 3.

Creek (1997b) Approaches to practice. In Creek J (Ed) Occupational Therapy and Mental Health, 2nd edn. Edinburgh: Churchill Livingstone, Ch. 5.

David A, Pelosi A, McDonald E, Stephens D, Ledger D, Rathbone R, Mann A (1990) Tired, weak, or in need of rest: fatigue among general practice attenders. British Medical Journal 301: 1199–1202.

David AS, Wessely S, Pelosi AJ (1988) Postviral fatigue syndrome: time for a new approach. British Medical Journal 296: 696–9.

Davies W (1993) Personal communication on taught course: Extended Training in Cognitive Therapy, Association of Psychological Therapies.

Deale A, Chalder T, Marks I, Wessely S (1997) Cognitive behaviour therapy for chronic fatigue syndrome: a randomised controlled trial. American Journal of Psychiatry 154(3): 408–14.

DeLuca J, Johnson SK, Natelson BH (1993) Information processing efficiency in chronic fatigue syndrome and multiple sclerosis. Archives of Neurology 50: 301–4.

DeLuca J, Johnson SK, Beldowicz D, Natelson BH (1995) Neuropsychological impairments in chronic fatigue syndrome, multiple sclerosis, and depression. Journal of Neurology, Neurosurgery and Psychiatry 58: 38–43.

DeLuca J, Johnson SK, Ellis PS, Natelson BH (1997) Cognitive functioning is impaired in patients with chronic fatigue syndrome devoid of psychiatric disease. Journal of Neurology, Neurosurgery and Psychiatry 62: 151–5.

Demitrack MA, Dale JK, Straus SE, Laue L, Listwak SJ, Kruesi MJP, Chrousos GP, Gold PW (1991) Evidence for impaired activation of the hypothalamic–pituitary–adrenal axis in patients with chronic fatigue syndrome. Journal of Clinical Endocrinology and Metabolism 73: 1224–34.

Denman AM (1990) The chronic fatigue syndrome: a return to common sense. Postgraduate Medical Journal 66: 499–501.

Deulofeu R, Gascon J, Gimenez N, Corachan M (1991) Magnesium and chronic fatigue syndrome (letter). Lancet 338: 641.

Dowsett EG, Ramsey AM, McCartney RA, Bell EJ (1990) Myalgic encephalomyelitis – a persistent enteroviral infection? Postgraduate Medical Journal 66: 526–30.

Eakin P (1989a) Assessments of activities of daily living: a critical review. British Journal of Occupational Therapy 52(1): 11–15.

Eakin P (1989b) Problems with assessments of activities of daily living. British Journal of Occupational Therapy 52(2): 50–4.

Eastwood AJ, Sheldon TA (1996) Organisation of asthma care: what difference does it make? A systematic review of the literature. Quality in Health Care 5(3): 134–43.

Edwards P, Jones S, Shale D, Thursz M (1996) Shared Care: A Model for Clinical Management. Oxford: Radcliffe Medical Press.

Ellis A (1962) Reason and Emotion in Psychotherapy. New York: Lyle Stuart.

Engel (1980) The clinical application of the biopsychosocial model. American Journal of Psychiatry 137(5): 535–44.

Enright SJ (1997) Cognitive behaviour therapy – clinical applications. British Medical Journal 314: 1811–16.

Epstein S, Katz L (1992) Coping ability, stress, productive load and symptoms. Journal of Personality and Social Psychology 62(5): 813–25.

Essame CS, Phelan S, Aggett P, White PD (1998) Pilot study of a multidisciplinary inpatient rehabilitation of severely incapacitated patients with chronic fatigue syndrome. Journal of Chronic Fatigue Syndrome 4(2): 51–60.

Euba R, Chalder T, Deale A, Wessely S (1996) A comparison of the characteristics of chronic fatigue syndrome in primary and tertiary care. British Journal of Psychiatry 168: 121–6.

Fisk JD, Ritvo PG, Ross L, Haase DA, Marrie TJ, Schlech WF (1994) Measuring the functional impact of fatigue: initial validation of the Fatigue Impact Scale. Clinical Infectious Diseases 18(Suppl 1): S79–83.

Fleming MH (1994) A commonsense practice in an uncommon world. In Mattingly C, Fleming MH (Eds) Clinical Reasoning: Forms of Inquiry in a Therapeutic Practice. Philadelphia: FA Davies, Ch. 5, pp. 94–115.

Fukuda K, Straus SE, Hickie I, Sharpe M, Dobbins JG, Komaroff A, and the International Chronic Fatigue Syndrome Study Group (1994) The chronic fatigue syndrome: a comprehensive approach to its definition and study. Annals of Internal Medicine 121: 953–9.

Fulcher K, White P (1996) A comparison of physiological and psychological parameters between CFS patients and healthy sedentary controls. Journal of Chronic Fatigue Syndrome 2: 148–9.

Fulcher KY, White PD (1997) Randomised controlled trial of graded exercise in patients with chronic fatigue syndrome. British Medical Journal 314: 1647–52.

Fulcher KY, White PD (1998) Chronic fatigue syndrome: a description of graded exercise treatment. Physiotherapy 84(5): 223–6.

Fuller NS, Morrison RE (1998) Chronic fatigue syndrome. Helping patients cope with this enigmatic illness. Postgraduate Medicine 103(1): 175–84.

Gantz N (1993) Management of a patient with chronic fatigue syndrome. In Dawson DM, Sabin TD (Eds) Chronic Fatigue Syndrome. Boston: Little, Brown, pp. 185–94.

Gantz NM (1991) Magnesium and chronic fatigue (letter). Lancet 338: 66.

Gantz NM, Holmes GP (1989) Treatment of patients with chronic fatigue syndrome. Drugs 38(6): 855–62.

Gibson H, Carroll N, Clague JE, Edwards RHT (1993) Exercise performance and fatiguability in patients with chronic fatigue syndrome. Journal of Neurology, Neurosurgery and Psychiatry 56: 993–8.

Gilliam (1992) The 1934 Los Angeles County Hospital Epidemic. In The Clinical and Scientific Basis of Myalgic Encephalomyelitis/Chronic Fatigue Syndrome. Ottawa: Nightingale Research Foundation, pp. 119–28.

Gold D, Bowden R, Sixbey J, Riggs R, Katon WJ, Ashley R, Obrigewitch R, Corey L (1990) Chronic fatigue: a prospective clinical and virologic study. Journal of the American Medical Association 264(1): 48–53.

Goldberg D, Williams P (1988) A User's Guide to the General Health Questionnaire. Windsor: NFER-Nelson.

Goldenberg DL, Felson DT, Dinerman H (1986) A randomised, controlled trial of amitriptyline and naproxen in the treatment of patients with fibromyalgia. Arthritis and Rheumatism 29(11): 1371–7.

Golledge (1998a) Distinguishing between occupation, purposeful activity and activity, part 1: review and explanation. British Journal of Occupational Therapy 61(3): 100–5.

Golledge (1998b) Distinguishing between occupation, purposeful activity and activity, part 2: why is the distinction important? British Journal of Occupational Therapy 61(4): 157–60.

Golledge (1998c) Is there unnecessary duplication of skills between occupational therapists and physiotherapists? British Journal of Occupational Therapy 61(4): 161–2.

Goodnick PJ, Sandoval R (1993) Psychotrophic treatment of chronic fatigue syndrome and related disorders. Journal of Clinical Psychiatry 54: 13–20.

Gow J, Behan P, Simpson K, McGarry F, Keir S (1994) Studies of enteroviruses in patients with chronic fatigue syndrome. Clinical Infectious Diseases 18(Suppl 1): S126–9.

Greenhalgh PM (1994) Shared Care for Diabetes: A Systematic Review. London: Royal College of General Practitioners.

Greenleaf JE, Kozlowski S (1982) Physiological consequences of reduced physical activity during bed rest. Exercise and Sports Sciences Review 10: 84–119.

Hagedorn R (1995) Occupational Therapy: Perspectives and Processes. London: Churchill Livingstone.

Hagedorn R (1997) Foundations for Practice in Occupational Therapy, 2nd edn. London: Churchill Livingstone.

Hall HJ (1905) The systematic use of work as a remedy in neurasthenia and allied conditions. Boston Medical and Surgical Journal 152(2): 29–32.

Halpin D, Wessely S (1989) VP-1 antigen in chronic postviral fatigue syndrome. Lancet 1(8645): 1028–9.

Hawton K, Salkovskis PM, Kirk J, Clark DM (Eds) (1989) Cognitive Behaviour Therapy for Psychiatric Problems. A Practical Guide. Oxford: Oxford University Press.

Henderson DA, Shelokov A (1959) Epidemic neuromyasthenia – clinical syndrome? In The Clinical and Scientific Basis of Myalgic Encephalomyelitis/Chronic Fatigue Syndrome. Ottawa: Nightingale Research Foundation (1992), pp. 159–75.

Hickie IB, Lloyd AR, Wakefield D, Parker G (1990) The psychiatric status of patients with chronic fatigue syndrome. British Journal of Psychiatry 156: 534–40.

Hickie IB, Lloyd AR, Hadzi-Pavlovic D, Parker G, Bird K, Wakefield D (1995) Can the chronic fatigue syndrome be defined by distinct clinical features? Psychological Medicine 25: 925–35.

Hickie IB, Lloyd AR, Wakefield D (1995) Chronic fatigue syndrome: current perspectives on evaluation and management. Medical Journal of Australia 163(6): 314–18.

Hinds GME, McCluskey DR (1993) A retrospective study of the chronic fatigue syndrome. Proceedings of the Royal College of Physicians of Edinburgh 23: 10–14.

Holloway F, Oliver N, Collins E, Carson J (1995) Case management: a critical review of the outcome literature. European Psychiatry 10(3): 113–28.

Holmes GP (1991) Defining the chronic fatigue syndrome. Reviews of Infectious Diseases 13(Suppl 1): S53–5.

Holmes GP, Kaplan JE, Gantz NM, Komaroff AL, Schonberger LB, Straus SE, Jones JF, Dubois RE, Cunningham-Rundles C, Pahwa S, Tosato G, Zegans LS, Purtilo DT, Brown N, Schoolet RT, Brus I (1988) Chronic fatigue syndrome: a working case definition. Annals of Internal Medicine 108: 387–9.

Ho-Yen Do (1990) Patient management of post-viral fatigue syndrome. British Journal of General Practitioners 40: 37–9.

Hughes SL, Ulasevich A, Weaver FM, Henderson W, Manheim L, Kubal JD, Bonarigo F (1997) Impact of home care on hospital days: a meta analysis. Health Services Research 32(4): 415–32.

Hyde BM (1992a) Myalgic encephalomyelitis (chronic fatigue syndrome): an historical perspective. In Hyde BM, Goldstein J, Levine P (Eds) The Clinical and Scientific Basis of Myalgic Encephalomyelitis/Chronic Fatigue Syndrome. Ottawa: Nightingale Research Foundation.

Hyde BM (1992b) The 1934 Los Angeles County Hospital epidemic. In Hyde BM, Goldstein J, Levine P (Eds) The Clinical and Scientific Basis of Myalgic Encephalomyelitis/Chronic Fatigue Syndrome. Ottawa: Nightingale Research Foundation.

Imboden JB, Canter A, Cluff LE (1961) Convalescence from influenza. A study of the psychological and clinical determinants. Archives of Internal Medicine 108: 393–9.

Jeffery LIH (1993) Aspects of selecting outcome measures to demonstrate the effectiveness of comprehensive rehabilitation. British Journal of Occupational Therapy 56(11): 394–400.

Jette A (1985) State of the art in functional status assessment. In Jules M Rothstein (Ed) Measurement in Physical Therapy. Edinburgh: Churchill Livingstone.

Johnson SK, DeLuca J, Natelson BH (1996) Personality dimensions in the chronic fatigue syndrome: a comparison with multiple sclerosis and depression. Journal of Psychiatric Research 30(1): 9–20.

Joyce E, Blumenthal S, Wessely S (1996) Memory, attention, and executive function in chronic fatigue syndrome. Journal of Neurology, Neurosurgery and Psychiatry 60: 495–503.

Joyce J, Wessely S (1996) Chronic fatigue syndrome. Irish Journal of Psychological Medicine 13(2): 46–50.

Joyce J, Hotopf M, Wessely S (1997) The prognosis of chronic fatigue and chronic fatigue syndrome: a systematic review. Quarterly Journal of Medicine 90: 223–33.

Karnofsky DA, Abelman WH, Craver LF, Burchenal JH (1948) The use of nitrogen mustards in the palliative treatment of carcinoma. Cancer 1: 634–56.

Kelly G (1995) Rights, ethics and the spirit of occupation (letter). British Journal of Occupational Therapy 58(2): 77–8.

Klug GA, McAuley E, Clark S (1989) Factors influencing the development and maintenance of aerobic fitness: lessons applicable to the fibrositis syndrome. Journal of Rheumatology 16(Suppl 19): 30–9.

Kormaroff A, Geiger AM (1988) IgG subclass deficiencies in chronic fatigue syndrome. Lancet 1(8597): 1288–9.

Kormaroff A, Geiger A (1989) Does the CDC working case definition of chronic fatigue syndrome (CFS) identify a distinct group? Clinical Research 37: 778A.

Kormaroff AL, Buchwald DS (1998) Chronic fatigue syndrome: an update. Annual Review of Medicine 49: 1–13.

Kroenke K, Wood DR, Mangelsdorff AD, Meier NJ, Powell JB (1988) Chronic fatigue in primary care. Prevalence, patient characteristics and outcome. Journal of the American Medical Association 260(7): 929–34.

Krupp LB, LaRocca NG, Muir-Nash J, Steinberg AD (1989) The Fatigue Severity Scale: application to patients with multiple sclerosis and systemic lupus erythematosus. Archives of Neurology 46: 1121–3.

Lambert R (1998) Occupation and lifestyle: implications for mental health practice. British Journal of Occupational Therapy 61(5): 193–7.

Lancet (1996) Editorial: Frustrating survey of chronic fatigue. Lancet 348: 971.

Lane TJ, Matthews DA, Manu P (1990) The low yield of physical examinations and laboratory investigations of patients with chronic fatigue. American Journal of Medical Sciences 299(5): 313–18.

Law M, Copper BA, Strong S, Stewart D, Rigby P, Letts L (1997) Theoretical contexts for the practice of occupational therapy. In Christiansen C, Baum C (Eds) Occupational Therapy: Enabling Function and Well Being, 2nd edn. New Jersey: Slack, Ch. 4.

Lazarus AA (1971) Behaviour Therapy and Beyond. New York: McGraw Hill.

Leibowitz MR, Quitkin FM, Stewart JW, McGrath PJ, Harrison WM, Markowitz JS, Rabkin JG, Tricamo E, Goetz DM, Klein DF (1988) Antidepressant specificity in atypical depression. Archives of General Psychiatry 45: 129–37.

Leitch AG (1994) The chronic fatigue syndrome reviewed. Proceedings of the Royal College of Physicians of Edinburgh 24: 480–508.

Levine PH, Snow PG, Ranum BA, Paul C, Holmes MJ (1997) Epidemic neuromyasthenia and chronic fatigue syndrome in West Otago, New Zealand. Archives of Internal Medicine 157: 750–4.

Lloyd AR, Wakefield A, Boughton C, Dwyer J (1988) What is myalgic encephalomyelitis? Lancet i: 1286–7.

Lloyd AR, Hickie I, Boughton CR, Spencer O, Wakefield D (1990a) Prevalence of chronic fatigue syndrome in an Australian population. Medical Journal of Australia 153: 522–8.

Lloyd AR, Hickie I, Wakefield D, Boughton C, Dwyer J (1990b) A double-blind, placebo-controlled trial of intravenous immunoglobulin therapy in patients with chronic fatigue syndrome. American Journal of Medicine 89: 561–8.

Lloyd AR, Gandevia SC, Hales JP (1991) Muscle performance, voluntary activation, twitch properties and perceived effort in normal subjects and patients with the chronic fatigue syndrome. Brain 114: 85–98.

Lloyd AR, Hickie I, Brockman A, Hickie C, Wilson A, Dwyer J, Wakefield D (1993) Immunologic and psychologic therapy for patients with chronic fatigue syndrome: a double-blind, placebo-controlled trial. American Journal of Medicine 94: 197–203.

Lynch S, Seth R (1989) Postviral fatigue syndrome and the VP-1 antigen. Lancet ii; 8672: 1160–1.

Lynch S, Seth R, Montgomery S (1991) Antidepressant therapy in chronic fatigue syndrome. British Journal of General Practitioners 41: 339–42.

Mahoney FI, Barthel DW (1965) Functional evaluation: the Barthel index. Maryland State Medical Journal 14: 61–3.

Main CJ (1983) The Modified Somatic Perception Questionnaire (MSPQ). Journal of Psychosomatic Research 27(6): 503–14.

Manu P, Matthews DA, Lane TJ (1988) The mental health of patients with a chief complaint of chronic fatigue. Archives of Internal Medicine 148: 2213–17.

Marshall PS, Forstot M, Callies A, Peterson PK, Schenck CH (1997) Cognitive slowing and working memory difficulties in chronic fatigue syndrome. Psychosomatic Medicine 59: 58–66.

Martin RM, Hilton SR, Kerry SM, Richards NM (1997) General practitioners' perceptions of the tolerability of antidepressant drugs: a comparison of selective serotonin reuptake inhibitors and tricyclic antidepressants. British Journal of Medicine 314: 646–51.

Matthews DA, Lane TJ, Manu P (1991) Antibodies to Epstein–Barr virus in patients with chronic fatigue. Southern Medical Journal 84(7): 832–40.

Mattingly C (1994) Occupational therapy as a two-body practice. In Clinical Reasoning: Forms of Inquiry in a Therapeutic Practice. Philadelphia: FA Davis, Ch. 4.

McCain GA, Bell DA, Mai FM, Halliday PD (1988) A controlled study of the effects of a supervised cardiovascular fitness training program on the manifestations of primary fibromyalgia. Arthritis and Rheumatism 31(9): 1135–41.

McCully KK, Sisto SA, Natelson BH (1996) Use of exercise for treatment of chronic fatigue syndrome. Sports Medicine 1: 35–48.

McDonald E, Cope H, David A (1993) Cognitive impairment in patients with chronic fatigue syndrome. Journal of Neurology, Neurosurgery and Psychiatry 56: 812–15.

McDonald E, David AS, Pelosi AJ, Mann AH (1993) Chronic fatigue in primary care attenders. Psychological Medicine 23: 987–98.

McEvedy CP, Beard AW (1970) Royal Free epidemic of 1955: a reconsideration. British Medical Journal i: 7.

McMahon R (1994) Trial and error: an experiment in practice. In Buckeldee J, McMahon R (Eds) The Research Experience in Nursing. London: Chapman & Hall.

Medical Outcomes Trust (1994) How to Score the SF-36 Health Survey. Boston, USA: Medical Outcomes Trust.

Moldofsky H (1995) Sleep, neuroimmune and neuroendocrine functions in fibromyalgia and chronic fatigue syndrome. Advances in Neuroimmunology 5: 39–56.

Morriss R, Sharpe M, Sharpley AL, Cowen PJ, Hawton K, Morris J (1993) Abnormalities of sleep in patients with the chronic fatigue syndrome. British Medical Journal 306: 1161–4.

Morriss R, Wearden AJ, Battersby L (1997) The relation of sleep difficulties to fatigue, mood and disability in chronic fatigue syndrome. Journal of Psychosomatic Research 42(6): 597–605.

Moss-Morris R, Petrie K, Large KJ, Kydd RR (1996) Neuropsychological deficits in chronic fatigue syndrome: artefact or reality? Journal of Neurology, Neurosurgery and Psychiatry 60: 474–7.

Natelson BH, Cheu J, Pareja J, Ellis SP, Policastro T, Findley TW (1996) Randomized, double blind, controlled placebo-phase in trial of low dose phenelzine in the chronic fatigue syndrome. Psychopharmacology 124: 226–30.

National Task Force on CFS/PVFS/ME (1994) Report. Bristol: Westcare.

National Task Force on CFS/ME (1998) NHS Services for People with Chronic Fatigue Syndrome/Myalgic Encephalomyelitis. Bristol: Westcare.

Nelson D (1997) Why the profession of occupational therapy will flourish in the 21st century. American Journal of Occupational Therapy 51(1): 11–24.

Ottenbacher KJ, Christainsen C (1997) Occupational performance assessment. In Christiansen C, Baum C (Eds) Occupational Therapy: Enabling Function and Well Being, 2nd edn. New Jersey: Slack, Ch. 5.

Parish JG (1978) Early outbreaks of 'epidemic neuromyasthenia'. Postgraduate Medical Journal 54: 711–17.

Paterson CF (1997) A short history of occupational therapy in mental health. In Creek J (Ed) Occupational Therapy and Mental Health. Edinburgh: Churchill Livingstone, Ch. 1.

Paterson CF (1998) Occupational therapy and the National Health Service, 1948–1998. British Journal of Occupational Therapy 61(7): 311–15.

Pawlikowska T, Chalder T, Hirsch SR, Wallace P, Wright DJM, Wessely SC (1994) Population based study of fatigue and psychological distress. British Medical Journal 308: 763–6.

Peel M (1988) Rehabilitation in postviral syndrome. Journal of Social Occupational Medicine 38: 44–5.

Pemberton S, Hatcher S, Stanley P, House A (1994) Chronic fatigue syndrome: a way forward. British Journal of Occupational Therapy 57(10): 381–3.

Peterson PK, Pheley A, Schroppel J, Schenck C, Marshall P, Kind A, Haugland JM, Lambrecht LJ, Swan S, Goldsmith S (1998) A preliminary placebo-controlled crossover trial of fludrocortisone for chronic fatigue syndrome. Archives of Internal Medicine 158: 908–14.

Petrie K, Moss-Morris R, Weinman J (1995) The impact of catastrophic beliefs on functioning in chronic fatigue syndrome. Journal of Psychosomatic Research 39(1): 31–7.

Piper B (1997) Measuring fatigue. In Frank-Stromborg M, Olsen SJ (Eds) Instruments for Clinical Health Care Research, 2nd edn. USA: Jones & Bartlett, pp. 482–96.

Prasher D, Smith A, Findley L (1990) Sensory and cognitive event-related potentials in myalgic encephalomyelitis. Journal of Neurology, Neurosurgery and Psychiatry 53: 247–53.

Ramsey AM (1978) 'Epidemic neuromyasthenia' 1955–1978. Postgraduate Medical Journal 54: 718–21.

Ray C, Weir WRC, Phillips S, Cullen S (1992a) Development of a measure of symptoms in chronic fatigue syndrome: the Profile of Fatigue-Related Symptoms (PFRS). Psychology and Health 7: 27–43.

Ray C, Weir WRC, Cullen S, Phillips S (1992b) Illness perception and symptom components in chronic fatigue syndrome. Journal of Psychosomatic Research 36(3): 243–56.

Ray C, Weir W, Stewart D, Miller P, Hyde G (1993) Ways of coping with chronic fatigue syndrome: development of an Illness Management Questionnaire (IMQ). Social Science and Medicine 37: 385–91.

Ray C, Jefferies S, Weir WRC (1995) Coping with chronic fatigue syndrome: illness responses and their relationship with fatigue, functional impairment and emotional status. Psychological Medicine 25: 937–45.

Ray C, Jefferies S, Weir W (1997) Coping and other predictors of outcome in chronic fatigue syndrome: a 1 year follow up. Journal of Psychosomatic Research 43(4): 405–15.

Ridsdale L, Evans A, Jerrett W, Mandalia S, Osler K, Vora H (1993) Patients with fatigue in general practice: a prospective study. British Medical Journal 307: 103–6.

Riley MS, O'Brien CJ, McCluskey DR, Bell NP, Nicholls DP (1990) Aerobic work capacity in patients with chronic fatigue syndrome. British Medical Journal 301: 953–6.

Rogers CR (1951) Client Centred Therapy: Its Current Practice, Implications and Theory. London: Constable.

Rossiter DA, Edmundson A, Al Shahi R, Thompson AJ (1998) Integrated care pathways in multiple sclerosis rehabilitation: completing the audit cycle. Multiple Sclerosis 4: 85–9.

Rowbottom D, Keast D, Pervan Z, Morton A (1998) The physiological response to exercise in chronic fatigue syndrome. Journal of Chronic Fatigue Syndrome 4(2): 33–49.

Royal Colleges of Physicians, General Practitioners and Psychiatrists (1996) Report: Chronic Fatigue Syndrome. London: Royal College of Physicians.

Russell-Hodgson C (1998) It's all good practice: linking primary care and social services in Greenwich. Journal of Interprofessional Care 12(1): 89–91.

Sabin TD, Dawson DM (1993) History and epidemiology. In Dawson DM, Sabin TD (Eds) Chronic Fatigue Syndrome. Boston: Little, Brown.

Salit IE (1997) Precipitating factors for the chronic fatigue syndrome. Journal of Psychiatric Research 31(1): 59–65.

Schluederberg A, Straus SE, Peterson P, Blumenthal S, Komaroff AL, Spring SB, Landay A, Buchwald D (1992) Chronic fatigue syndrome research. Definition and medical outcome assessment. Annals of Internal Medicine 117(4): 325–31.

Schwartz JE, Jandorf L, Krupp LB (1993) The measurement of fatigue: a new instrument. Journal of Psychosomatic Research 37(7): 753–62.

Sharpe M, Wessely S (1998) Putting the rest cure to rest – again: rest has no place in treating chronic fatigue. British Journal of Medicine 316: 796.

Sharpe M (1991) Psychiatric management of PVFS. British Medical Bulletin 47(4): 989–1005.

Sharpe M (1998) Cognitive behaviour therapy. In Fox R (Ed) for The Linbury Trust A Research Portfolio on Chronic Fatigue. London: Royal Society of Medicine.

Sharpe MC, Archard LC, Banatvala JE, Borysiewicz JE, Clare AW, David A, Edwards RHT, Hawton KEH, Lambert HP, Lane RJM, McDonald EM, Mowbray JF, Pearson DJ, Peto TEA, Preddy VR, Smith AP, Smith DG, Taylor DJ, Tyrell DAJ, Wessely S, White PD (1991) A report – chronic fatigue syndrome: guidelines for research. Journal of the Royal Society of Medicine 84: 118–21.

Sharpe M, Hawton K, Seagroatt V, Pasvol G (1992) Follow up of patients presenting with fatigue to an infectious diseases clinic. British Medical Journal 305: 147–52.

Sharpe M, Hawton K, Simkin S, Surawy C, Hackman A, Klimes I, Peto T, Warrell D, Seagrott V (1996) Cognitive behaviour therapy for the chronic fatigue syndrome: a randomised controlled trial. British Medical Journal 312: 22–6.

Sharpe M, Chalder T, Palmer I, Wessely S (1997) Chronic fatigue syndrome: a practical guide to assessment and management. General Hospital Psychiatry 19: 185–99.

Sharpley A, Clements A, Hawton K, Sharpe M (1997) Do patients with 'pure' chronic fatigue syndrome (neurasthenia) have abnormal sleep? Psychosomatic Medicine 59: 592–6.

Shefer A, Dobbins JG, Fukuda K, Steele L, Koo D, Nisenbaum R, Rutherford GW (1997) Fatiguing illness among employees in three large state office buildings, California 1993: was there an outbreak? Journal of Psychiatric Research 31(1): 31–43.

Sigurdsson B, Gudmundsson KR (1956) Clinical findings six years after outbreak of Akureyri disease. Lancet i: 766.

Simons AD, Murphy GE, Levine JL, Wetzel RD (1986) Cognitive therapy and pharmacotherapy for depression. Archives of General Psychiatry 43: 43–8.

Stewart A, Hays RD, Ware J (1988) The MOS short form general health survey. Medical Care 26: 724–35.

Straus SE (1992) Defining the chronic fatigue syndrome. Archives of Internal Medicine 152: 1569–70.

Straus SE (1996) Chronic fatigue syndrome: biopsychosocial approach may be difficult in practice. British Medical Journal 313: 831–2.

Surawy C, Hackman A, Hawton K, Sharpe M (1995) Chronic fatigue syndrome: a cognitive approach. Behavioural Research and Therapy 33(5): 535–44.

Swanink CMA, Vercoulen JHMM, Bleijenberg G, Fennis JFM, Galama JMD, Van Der Meer JWM (1995) Chronic fatigue syndrome: a clinical and laboratory study with a well matched control group. Journal of Internal Medicine 237: 499–506.

Tanner D (1998) Empowerment and care management: swimming against the tide. Health and Social Care in the Community 6(6): 447–57.

Thomas PK (1993) The chronic fatigue syndrome: what do we know? British Medical Journal 306: 1557–8.

Valdini A, Steinhardt S, Feldman E (1989) Usefulness of a standard battery of laboratory tests in investigating chronic fatigue in adults. Family Practice 6(4): 286–91.

Vercoulen JHMM, Swanink CMA, Fennis JFM, Galama JMD, Van der Meer LWM, Bleijenberg G (1994) Dimensional assessment of chronic fatigue syndrome. Journal of Psychosomatic Research 38(5): 383–92.

Vercoulen JHMM, Swanink CMA, Fennis JFM, Galama JMD, Van der Meer LWM, Bleijenberg G (1996) Prognosis in chronic fatigue syndrome: a prospective study on the natural course. Journal of Neurology, Neurosurgery and Psychiatry 60: 489–94.

Vercoulen JHMM, Bazelmans E, Swanink CMA, Fennis JFM, Galama JMD, Jongen PJH, Hommes O, Van der Meer JWM, Bleijenberg G (1997) Physical activity in chronic fatigue syndrome: assessment and its role in fatigue. Journal of Psychiatric Research 31(6): 661–73.

Vollmer-Conna U, Hickie I, Hadzi-Pavlovic D, Tymms K, Wakefield D, Lloyd A (1997) Intravenous immunoglobulin is ineffective in the treatment of patients with chronic fatigue syndrome. American Journal of Medicine 103: 38–43.

Wagenmakers AJM, Coakley JH, Edwards RHT (1988) The metabolic consequences of reduced habitual activities in patients with muscle pain and disease. Ergonomics 31(11): 1519–27.

Wallace PG (1991) Epidemiology: a critical review. British Medical Bulletin 47(4): 942–51.

Ware JE, Sherborne CD (1992) The MOS 36-item Short Form Health Survey (SF-36). Conceptual framework and item selection. Medical Care 30(6): 473–83.

Ware JE, Snow KK, Kosinski M, Gandek B (1993) SF-36 Health Survey. Manual and Interpretation Guide. Boston: Health Institute.

Wearden A, Appleby L (1997) Cognitive performance and complaints of cognitive impairment in chronic fatigue syndrome (CFS). Psychological Medicine 27: 81–90.

Wearden AJ, Morris RK, Mullis R, Strickland PL, Pearson DJ, Appleby L, Campbell IT, Morris JA (1998) A randomised, double blind, placebo controlled treatment trial of fluoxetine and a graded exercise programme in chronic fatigue syndrome. British Journal of Psychiatry 172: 485–90.

Wessely S (1989) Myalgic encephalomyelitis – a warning: discussion paper. Journal of the Royal Society of Medicine 82: 215–17.

Wessely S (1990) Old wine in new bottles: neurasthenia and 'ME'. Psychological Medicine 20: 35–53.

Wessely S (1991) History of postviral fatigue syndrome. British Medical Bulletin 47(4): 919–41.

Wessely S (1992) Chronic fatigue syndrome: current issues. Reviews of Medical Microbiology 3: 211–16.

Wessely S (1995a) The epidemiology of chronic fatigue syndrome. Epidemiologic Reviews 17: 139–51.

Wessely S (1995b) Chronic fatigue syndrome – the current position, 1: Background, epidemiology and aetiology. Primary Care Psychiatry 1: 21–30.

Wessely S (1995c) Cognitive behaviour therapy and chronic fatigue syndrome. Why? In: Demitrack M, Abbey S (Eds) Chronic Fatigue Syndrome: Psychiatric and Practical Issues. New York: Guilford Press.

Wessely S, Powell R (1989) Fatigue syndromes: a comparison of chronic 'post viral' fatigue with neuromuscular and affective disorder. Journal of Neurology, Neurosurgery and Psychiatry 52: 940–8.

Wessely S, Thomas PK (1990) The chronic fatigue syndrome – myalgic encephalomyelitis or postviral fatigue. In Recent Advances in Clinical Neurology, 6. Edinburgh: Churchill Livingstone.

Wessely S, David A, Butler S, Chalder T (1989) Management of chronic (post viral) fatigue syndrome. Journal of the Royal College of General Practitioners 39: 26–9.

Wessely S, Chalder T, Hirsch S, Pawlikowska T, Wallace P, Wright DJM (1995) Post-infectious fatigue: prospective cohort study in primary care. Lancet 345: 1333–8.

Wessely S, Chalder T, Hirsch S, Wallace P, Wright D (1996) Psychological symptoms, somatic symptoms, and psychiatric disorder in chronic fatigue and chronic fatigue syndrome: a prospective study in the primary care setting. American Journal of Psychiatry 153: 1050–9.

Wessely S, Hotopf M, Sharpe M (1998) Chronic Fatigue and its Syndromes. Oxford: Oxford University Press, pp. 363, 386, 387.

White PD, Cleary KJ (1997) An open study of the efficacy and adverse effects of moclobemine in patients with the chronic fatigue syndrome. International Clinical Psychopharmacology 12: 47–52.

White PD, Thomas JM, Amess J, Grover SA, Kangro HO, Clare AW (1995) The existence of a fatigue syndrome after glandular fever. Psychological Medicine 25: 907–16.

Wilcox AA (1998) Occupation for health. British Journal of Occupational Therapy 61(8): 340–5.

Willians AC de C, Nicholas MK, Richardson PH, Pither CE, Justins DM, Chamberlain JH, Harding VR, Ralphs JA, Jones SC, Dieudonne I, Featherstone JD, Hodgson DR, Ridout KL, Shannon EM (1993) Evaluation of a cognitive behavioural programme for rehabilitating patients with chronic pain. British Journal of General Practice 43: 513–18.

Wilson A, Hickie I, Lloyd A, Hadzi-Pavlovic D, Boughton C, Dwyer J, Wakefield D (1994a) Longitudinal study of outcome of chronic fatigue syndrome. British Medical Journal 308: 756–9.

Wilson A, Hickie I, Lloyd A, Wakefield D (1994b) The treatment of chronic fatigue syndrome: science and speculation. American Journal of Medicine 96: 544–50.

Wood C, Magnello ME, Sharpe MC (1992) Fluctuations in perceived energy and mood among patients with chronic fatigue syndrome. Journal of the Royal Society of Medicine 85: 195–8.

Yeomans JDI, Conway SP (1991) Biopsychosocial aspects of chronic fatigue syndrome (myalgic encephalomyelitis). Journal of Infection 23: 263–9.

Young AH, Sharpe M, Clements A, Dowling B, Hawton KE, Cowen PJ (1998) Basal activity of the hypothalamic–pituitary–adrenal axis in patients with chronic fatigue syndrome (neurasthenia). Biological Psychiatry 43: 236–7.

Yousef G, Bell E, Mann G, Muru-Gesan V, Smith DG, McCarthey RA, Mowbray JF (1988)
    Chronic enterovirus infection in patients with postviral fatigue syndrome. Lancet i
    (8578): 146–50.
Zigmond AS, Snaith RP (1983) The Hospital Anxiety and Depression Scale. Acta
    Psychiatrica Scandinavica 67: 361–70.

Appendix 1:
Booklets Given Following Occupational Therapy Sessions

(Reproduced with the kind permission of Havering Hospitals NHS Trust)

Havering Hospitals NHS Trust:
Booklet Number One
What is Chronic Fatigue Syndrome?

© CFS Team, Havering Hospitals NHS Trust, 1996
First produced by Diane Cox, 1994

> Adapted from an original idea by Dr Simon Hatcher
> Leeds Fatigue Clinic
> Seacroft Hospital
> Leeds LS14 6UH

Chronic Fatigue Syndrome Diagnostic and Management Service
Essex Centre for Neurological Sciences
Oldchurch Hospital
Romford, Essex RM7 0BE

What is Chronic Fatigue Syndrome (CFS)?

Chronic fatigue syndrome (CFS) is a condition which can affect people in a variety of ways. A number of names have been used to describe this syndrome, such as myalgic encephalomyelitis (ME) and post-viral fatigue syndrome but the consensus at present suggests that chronic fatigue syndrome is the most appropriate title as it identifies the most predominant feature: fatigue.

The main complaint is persistent fatigue, which differs from normal tiredness. The fatigue is usually severe and disabling, affecting physical and mental functioning. It is often accompanied by a range of other unpleasant symptoms such as muscle and/or joint pain, headache, poor concentration, memory difficulties and many others. Problems with sleep

143

are common and include sleeping longer than normal or having difficulty getting off to sleep and waking frequently. Whatever the problem the sleep is seldom refreshing.

How is it Diagnosed?

At present no specific diagnostic test is available and diagnosis is made with reference to the symptoms and through clinical evaluation to exclude any other cause for fatigue. This will mean having several blood tests and perhaps a head scan (CT scan), X-rays and an EEG. Prof. Findley will have arranged these through clinic, whilst you are an inpatient, or through your GP.

What Causes Chronic Fatigue Syndrome?

There is no one theory on the actual cause of chronic fatigue syndrome. The current thinking is that different causes or *triggers* start the illness, resulting in the same outcome of chronic fatigue.

The main triggers that have been identified are viral infections, internal and external stress and overwork. However, people have also noted *Candida*, allergies and diet. For most people it is a combination of these factors.

The scientific evidence now suggests that a part of the brain called the hypothalamic–pituitary–adrenal axis is affected. This particular part of the brain affects our internal control system (autonomic system), which is why people can have such a variety of symptoms and problems e.g. mood changes, nausea, dizziness, tinnitus, temperature control, sleep disturbance, anxiety and breathing changes.

How Chronic Fatigue Syndrome Affects Daily Life

The types of activities that result in increased fatigue will vary from person to person but will affect daily living. The types of activities which can be affected are: getting washed and dressed, reading a book, going to the shops, preparing a meal, talking or writing to friends and family, all of which can become exhausting.

The advice given to patients can be misleading; patients are often told to 'rest until the symptoms subside' or to 'learn to live within your limits', both of which will have different meanings for different people. This advice leads to further inactivity, as following rest any physical effort can increase the symptoms of fatigue and pain. Activity then starts to be avoided. The person will then have increased his/her sensitivity to any stimulation (mental or physical activity) and therefore tend to carry out little or no activity to avoid increased symptoms. Demoralization and low mood are often understandable consequences of the illness owing to the degree of disruption caused to everyday life. People often find themselves caught in a seesaw pattern of rest and activity or peaks and troughs that are determined by the presence or absence of symptoms and which are controlled by mood, fears and beliefs.

In the same way as the illness will have been triggered by certain factors there will be *perpetuators* of your illness that need to be identified. These will be similar, usually stress and recurrent infections, and there are patterns that can develop in response to the symptoms (see Booklet 2).

Duration and Treatment

A person with chronic fatigue syndrome will not recover by merely resting *or* by pushing him/herself to the absolute limit. Strenuous activity following prolonged periods of rest has been shown to increase symptoms, which perpetuates and reinforces activity-avoidance behaviour. Conversely, in a well phase people will tend to push themselves beyond their capacity in an attempt to regain 'normal' function. A variety of lifestyle management techniques will be used over the next few weeks to enable you to improve your level of ability.

The techniques will be used in conjunction with any medication Prof. Findley or your GP has prescribed for you. The drugs you are taking may vary within the group; this is because not all drugs react the same for each person. The types of drugs used will be those that react with the brain transmitters, such as antidepressants. The amount of time you have had the illness may differ from others in the group; the shortest duration will be six months. The average duration of the illness is four years. It is impossible to tell accurately how long your illness will last, but most people make a full recovery in time.

The overall purpose of treatment is to enable an increase in sustained activity on a daily basis using the principles and practice of graded activity and cognitive behaviour therapy.

Havering Hospitals NHS Trust:
Booklet Number Two
Graded Activity: What It Is and How to Do It

First produced by Diane Cox, 1994
  Adapted from an original idea by Dr Simon Hatcher
                          Leeds Fatigue Clinic
                          Seacroft Hospital
                          Leeds LS14 6UH

Chronic Fatigue Syndrome Diagnostic and Management Service
Essex Centre for Neurological Sciences
Oldchurch Hospital
Romford, Essex RM7 0BE

What is Graded Activity ?

Graded activity is a simple method of planning your activities and gradually increasing what you do. It is *not* an exercise programme!! It aims to give you control over your illness rather than the fatigue controlling you.

What are the Effects of Rest?

Although rest is an effective way of reducing tiredness and brings symptom relief in the short term, in the long term it is less helpful as it reduces exercise tolerance and can produce increased weakness, muscle wasting, cardiac and respiratory difficulties and increased sensitivity to activity. Prolonged rest brings about short-term symptom reduction but a long-term increase in disability. Following a period of rest, any activity produces an increase in a range of associated symptoms.

This results in a vicious circle of fluctuating bursts of activity and rest as people try to control and manage the illness by responding to the symptoms. This is called peaks and troughs. People end up alternating between doing too much on a good day (well phase) – *peak* – and then too little on a bad day (poor phase) – *trough* – in order to recover and reduce symptoms, leaving themselves in a physiological and psychological limbo (see handouts used during occupational therapy sessions).

Excessive rest may mean that you are not achieving anything, so you feel a failure compared with what you used to do. It may also mean you have more time on your hands to brood on your condition and become frustrated and bored.

Is Activity Harmful?

Graded activity is not about exercise but about daily life and lifestyle management. Most people, when they start grading their activity, actually have to cut down rather than add in activity!! Graded activity does not mean pushing beyond your limits. It aims to stop the peak–trough cycle and replace it with a *gradual* change in your daily routine.

Where Do I Start ?

The initial stage is to build up a picture of exactly how much activity is carried out on a daily basis, in particular your pattern of rest, activity and symptoms. Once this is established we can plan strategies to enable gradual and systematic increase in the amount of activity in a step-by-step fashion. The steps (goals/targets) need to be realistic and achievable.

Scheduling Activity and Rest

Pacing is the key. Graded activity aims to enable sustained and consistent activity on a daily basis. Doing tasks in stages and slowly building up how much you can do takes time, however this will help you to achieve more in the long run and sustain it. Goals or steps are established that concentrate on each person's major difficulties. The purpose of these goals is to facilitate:

(1) a gradual increase in tolerance to activity;
(2) a reduction in symptoms;
(3) an increase in previously avoided behaviours and activities.

The major problem people encounter on returning to activity is that if they were previously very fit and active they are more likely to attempt a rapid return to high levels of activity/exercise to which the body cannot respond due to its physical decondition. Activity has to be paced and gradual. Also, people will tend in a good phase to do all the activity they have not been able to do in a bad phase in an attempt to catch up.

Rest needs to be timetabled into each day, regardless of symptoms, so that it becomes consistent and part of the daily routine rather than varying dependent upon symptoms. For some people it helps initially to structure each day to gain an understanding of the balance required between rest and effort (see Figure 1: Daily programme example).

This amount of structure will not be required for all people; however, both rest and activity need to be scheduled into each day regardless of symptoms being present or not. During the session(s) you will select goals which are important to you. We will then consider these and timetable them into your daily life. You will need to break each goal down into achievable tasks.

Chronic fatigue syndrome:

Date:......................... Name:..................................

Time	Activity
9:00 am	Wake up/activity session
10:00 am	Rest period
10:30 am	Activity session
12:00 noon	Rest period
12:30 pm	Activity session
2:30 pm	Rest period
3:30 pm	Activity session
5:30 pm	Rest period
6:00 pm	Activity session
8:00 pm	Rest period
8:30 pm	Activity session
9:30 pm	$\frac{1}{2}$ hour wind down
10:00 pm	Bed

Figure 1

The goals are clear and specific, and set at a manageable level. They are increased gradually to slowly increase the amount of activity carried out each day. Examples of goals people have set themselves include:

(1) To get up at 9:00 am every day.
(2) To walk for 15 minutes three times a day.
(3) To rest for half an hour five times a day.
(4) To have a friend visit twice a week.
(5) To go to the supermarket once a week.

What to Expect

Initially when carrying out activity on a daily basis at a level you can manage, there will be a temporary increase in fatigue and other symptoms. It is important to expect this, but to realize that it will be only temporary. It does not mean that the treatment is not working, or that the illness is worse – it is just that your body needs to get used to this new pattern of planned, consistent activity and rest. It is important to persevere with your chosen tasks/targets as once your body becomes used to the pattern, the symptoms will subside by themselves, and you will be able to move onto the next stage.

Difficulty with Mental Tasks

Many chronic fatigue syndrome patients lose their ability to distinguish between important and unimportant sensations. This is why you may have difficulty shopping. Information bombards your ears and eyes resulting in *sensory overload* and fatigue. Normally when we shop we pay attention only to the information that is relevant, for example the prices, and would automatically screen out other information such as the presence of other people or the noise. People with chronic fatigue syndrome give the same importance to all these sensations which then compete for attention – it is not surprising they get tired!! Management of the sensory overload is just as important as physical management, and for some people is the *most* important aspect of the daily management of chronic fatigue syndrome.

Techniques for Memory and Concentration

(1) *Keep lists*
- This aids memory by repetition. The written list acts as a reminder as well as helping you pace your activities.
- Keep the lists short, three to four items at the most. This way you are less likely to forget part of the list.
(2) *Identify the times when you are more mentally alert* and keep mental tasks for those times. This may not always be possible. Remember: try to avoid mental tasks just prior to bed, as this may increase your difficulty getting off to sleep.
(3) When you are completing a task that needs concentration, *cut down on competing sensations*. For example, if you are driving, switch off the radio and ask any passengers not to talk.
(4) When reading, some people find it helpful to have a *reading window* to limit distractions. This is simply one or two pieces of paper, preferably white, to show only one/two lines at a time. As you read you move the card down the page. What this does is block out competing information from the rest of the page. This idea can be taken further by reading on a table cleared of all other material – again this removes competing information.
(5) *Use mnemonics* (memory tricks) to remember things. For example,

use the first letter of each word you need to remember and make up a smaller word, i.e. NATO = North Atlantic Treaty Organisation. Or link items with locations or places; for example, when introduced to someone new link their name with a county or country.

(6) *Games* can be helpful in improving memory and concentration. They are mental exercises, so the same rules apply as to activity. 'Start simple' for short periods, and gradually build up. Crosswords help verbal skills; computer games or cards help non-verbal skills. You can create your own games by reading part of the paper or an article, and then getting someone to ask you questions about it. Remember: keep it short and simple to start with.

Summary

(1) Plan your time.
(2) Plan rest and relaxation periods into each day.
(3) Break each activity into smaller manageable and achievable stages.
(4) Carry out the same amount of activity and rest every day.
(5) Avoid over-activity when you are feeling good or enthusiastic and reducing activity when you are feeling bad.
(6) Increase activity and reduce rest slowly and gradually.
(7) Don't expect to feel better immediately; remember that your immediate goal is to stick to the programme, not to overcome all your symptoms.
(8) If you work steadily at becoming more active, you will eventually find your symptoms resolving.

Havering Hospitals NHS Trust: Booklet Number Three

Rest, Relaxation and Stress: Learning to Relax and Manage Stress

© CFS Team, Havering Hospitals NHS Trust, 1996
First produced by Diane Cox, 1994

> Adapted from an original idea by Dr Simon Hatcher
> Leeds Fatigue Clinic
> Seacroft Hospital, Leeds LS14 6UH

Chronic Fatigue Syndrome Diagnostic and Management Service
Essex Centre for Neurological Sciences
Oldchurch Hospital
Romford, Essex RM7 0BE

Rest and Relaxation

Throughout daily life, *activity* needs to be balanced with *rest*. We cannot function without adequate rest. Rest can mean different things to different people. Some people may suggest that rest means sleeping or perhaps just sitting down and 'not doing anything'. Others may suggest that rest means being able to relax. When the term rest is used in your individual programme it means *relaxation*.

What is Relaxation?

Prior to becoming ill you may have found reading, watching TV or talking to friends on the telephone a good way to unwind. Now, however, due to the 'overactive brain' or 'sensory overload' phenomena (explained in Booklet 2) experienced in CFS/ME, the concept of relaxation needs to be redefined.

Anything that stimulates or over-stimulates the brain in terms of either physical or mental effort is termed *activity*. Thus talking, watching TV, reading and even eating are regarded as activities. Relaxation should focus not just on resting the body, but also on resting the mind.

Relaxation aims to achieve a state of minimal neurological (brain) activity. On a continuum between wakefulness and sleep X indicates the point at which relaxation occurs.

Asleep ◄——X————————————————► Awake

It is important *not* to go to sleep during a relaxation session. The only exception is the use of relaxation to assist with sleep at the end of the day. As you begin to implement the techniques you may well find that your sleep patterns improve, owing to a more helpful balance of *rest* and *activity* throughout the day.

What is Recreation?

Recreational activities are what you may have previously described as relaxation. These are 'the stress relievers', for example going to the pub after a busy day at work to unwind, playing a game of tennis, watching TV, gardening. In the main, they tend to be the activities you find enjoyable and that give you pleasure. Recreational activities are important in daily life and will, in time, need to be reintroduced as part of your programme of rest and activity

What is Stress ?

Stress can be anything that disturbs your status quo. This can be mental or physical. When this happens your body reacts in various ways to try to restore its balance and you may experience a variety of symptoms.

What are Stressful Events ?

A stressful event can be anything that you perceive as threatening: change in your life or disturbing emotions. Examples could include a car crash, divorce, moving house, prolonged difficult relationships, bringing up children alone, change of role in the home, examinations, work pressure, overwork. The list is endless. The actual event triggering stress will depend on the individual, but the most important thing is to be able to identify it and to recognize its effects on the body.

What Reaction Does the Stress Cause?

The body's first reaction to stress is a surge of adrenaline and steroids. This prepares the body for a 'flight or fight reaction'. For example, if you narrowly miss having an accident you may feel tense, sweaty, have a dry mouth and your heart rate increases. The feeling goes away if the stress is removed.

If the stress does not go away – for example continuing arguments with a partner or child, or a busy lifestyle or a chronic illness – then the early reactions can become permanent. If stress continues for a long time, the body becomes unable to maintain its balance and may 'break down'. This may take the form of chronic conditions such as migraine, high blood pressure and stomach upsets.

What Role Does Stress Play in Chronic Fatigue Syndrome?

Stress may be involved in two ways:

(1) It may help to cause or trigger the illness. For example, people under stress are more vulnerable to infections. This is because stress alters your body's immune system.
(2) Once the syndrome is established stress may be the cause of some of the symptoms. Certain complaints such as nervousness, muscle tension – especially in the neck region and upper spine, palpitations and sweating are all symptoms common in chronic fatigue syndrome.

What Can I Do About Stress?

There are two things you can do:

(1) You can try to identify and remove sources of stress in your life.
(2) You can help your body to maintain its balance and prevent symptoms of stress. This can be done in various ways. These include learning the difference between recreation and relaxation, and the importance of effective relaxation through the use of techniques such as breathing exercises and relaxation.

How to Relax

Creating a feeling of relaxation incorporates being able to 'switch off' both physically and mentally. There are a number of strategies you can use to help you to achieve this. For example:

(1) breathing exercises;
(2) listening to soft relaxation music;
(3) following a guided relaxation technique.

However, relaxation is a skill. It needs to be learnt. Initially the aim is to relax in a quiet environment where you feel comfortable and free from distraction. Once established, the techniques can be used in alternative environments; for example, at work, on the bus etc.

Why is it Important to Control My Breathing?

Stress can cause your breathing pattern to alter. You may begin to breathe more quickly, taking shallow breaths – this is called *hyperventilating*. If the stress is prolonged, hyperventilating may become a habit and you may not even be aware of your new breathing pattern. This may cause or exacerbate some of the symptoms of chronic fatigue syndrome. A quick test to see if you are hyperventilating is to try to hold your breath. If you cannot hold your breath for more than 10 seconds then you may be hyperventilating.

Many of the symptoms of hyperventilation are caused by overbreathing. This causes the blood chemistry to alter, which then produces symptoms such as chest pain, palpitations, anxiety and panic. In turn, these symptoms are a new source of stress and cause more hyperventilation. A vicious circle then starts. If you can control the depth and pace of your breathing and so stop these symptoms, you can begin to relax. The following are some examples of breathing exercises and relaxation techniques you can try.

How Can I Control My Breathing?

First, be *aware* of your breathing. The following procedure will help you become more aware of how you are breathing. You can do this sitting, standing or lying.

* Place one hand on the top of your chest.
* Place your other hand at the bottom of your rib cage, over the triangle formed where your ribs separate.
* Breathe normally and see which hand moves the most.
* If the top hand moves the most then your breathing is likely to be shallow, using only your upper chest and associated with stress.
* If the bottom hand moves more then you are breathing using your diaphragm, which means your breathing is deep, and your lungs are filling with air. This is associated with relaxation.

Abdominal (Diaphragmatic) Breathing Exercise

(1) Note the amount of tension you are feeling, then place one hand on your abdomen right beneath your rib cage.
(2) Inhale slowly and deeply through your nose into the 'bottom' of your lungs – in other words send the air as low as you can. If you are breathing from your abdomen, your hand will rise. Your chest should move only slightly while your abdomen expands.
(3) When you have taken in a full breath, pause for a moment and then breathe out slowly through your nose or mouth, depending on your preference. Be sure to exhale fully. As you exhale, allow your whole body to just let go. (Picture your arms and legs going loose and limp like a rag doll.)
(4) Do 10 slow full abdominal breaths. Try to keep your breathing smooth and regular, without gulping in a big breath, or letting your breath out all at once. Remember to pause briefly at the end of each inhalation. Count to 10, progressing with each exhalation.

The process should go like this:

Slow inhale........ Pause....... Slow exhale – count 1
Slow inhale........ Pause....... Slow exhale – count 2
Slow inhale........ Pause....... Slow exhale – count 3

and so on up to 10. If you start to feel light headed whilst practising abdominal breathing, stop for 30 seconds while you breathe normally and then start again.

Five minutes of abdominal breathing will have a pronounced impact in reducing anxiety or early symptoms of panic.

How Long Should I Do Breathing Exercises For?

Breathing exercises are aimed at giving you control over your breathing. Once this is achieved you should return to your natural breathing rhythms. If you continue to concentrate on your breathing you will become 'over aware' of it and this could bring back the feelings of stress. *Only do controlled breathing exercises for a maximum of 10 minutes twice a day.*

Benson's Relaxation

Find a comfortable position, sitting, lying or standing. Close eyes.

Stage One

- Breathe normally, in and out. Find your own natural rhythm.
- Continue to breathe normally for approximately 30 seconds.
- Take one deep breath, hold briefly and exhale. Breathe in through your nose and out through your mouth.
- Return to normal breathing for about 30 seconds.

Stage Two

- Still breathing normally, each time you breathe out say to yourself the word *smooth*. Just say the word to yourself in your head. As an alternative find another word that symbolizes or creates a sense of relaxation for example: *peace* or *calm*.
- Do this for about 30–40 seconds.

Stage Three

- Still continuing to breathe normally, now take on a 'passive attitude'.
- What this means is that nothing matters for five minutes: no sounds,

thoughts, voices, noises. *Nothing* matters for five minutes.
• To help you do this, allow yourself to hear a sound whether near or far, acknowledge the sound and then let it go.

On completion of the relaxation spend some time enjoying the feeling; never get up or move too quickly afterwards.

Points to Remember About Relaxation

(1) Start learning in a comfortable position, such as semi-lying or sitting. If possible choose a quiet place free from distractions. Pull the curtains, dim the lights or wear an eye mask.
(2) Make sure you are warm, as body temperature can dip during relaxation.
(3) Try to keep to the regular times suggested.
(4) Think about your breathing, try to breathe deeply and slowly. Observe your body, take notice when it tells you it is tense or relaxed.
(5) *Enjoy it*!!

Havering Hospitals NHS Trust: Booklet Number Four

Healthy Living: The Importance of Improving Sleep, Healthy Eating and Introducing Appropriate Levels of Exercise

© CFS Team, Havering Hospitals NHS Trust, 1997
First produced by Diane Cox, 1994

Booklet adapted from an original idea by Dr Simon Hatcher (1993–94)
Leeds Fatigue Clinic
Seacroft Hospital, Leeds LS14 6UH

Chronic Fatigue Syndrome Diagnostic and Management Service
Essex Centre for Neurological Sciences
Oldchurch Hospital
Romford, Essex RM7 0BE

How to Improve Your Sleep

Difficulty sleeping is frequently a problem in chronic fatigue syndrome and you have probably found that your sleep is not nearly as refreshing as it was before you became ill. Common difficulties include sleeping too much, difficulty falling asleep and broken sleep. Sleep patterns can also become disrupted, from taking catnaps during the day to being awake all night and asleep during the daytime.

There are several factors that can influence sleep and can contribute to irregular sleep patterns: daytime inactivity, daytime catnaps, inability to get to sleep at night.

Drinking too much coffee and tea can cause difficulty with sleep. They both contain caffeine, which is a stimulant and can keep you awake. Try to change to decaffeinated coffee and tea if you have sleep problems and limit your intake to three cups of coffee a day or five cups of tea. It may be helpful not to drink caffeinated beverages after mid-afternoon. Try drinking more mineral water, fruit juice or herb/fruit teas.

As you gradually increase your activity and reduce rest, you should notice an improvement in your sleep pattern. However, sometimes when the abnormal or broken sleep has become habitual, it can be difficult for your body to return to a normal pattern. You may find it helpful to tackle your sleep directly.

(1) Establish a Routine

Get up at the same time each morning irrespective of what time you fell asleep the night before. If you are tending to sleep too much or long into the day, gradually cut back by getting up earlier, in half-hour or hour blocks, i.e. 11:00 am instead of 12:00 noon until you reach your target time. Starting a new routine may make you feel more tired initially, but in a short time you will find yourself adjusting to it and feeling more energetic. In other words, although you may not be getting the same quantity of sleep, the quality will improve.

(2) Prepare for Sleep

Avoid activities which will keep you alert such as studying, work-related projects, decision making and include some sort of relaxation, such as having a warm bath or doing a relaxation exercise. Develop a routine before going to bed which will act as a signal for your body that it is preparing for sleep such as locking up, brushing teeth.

(3) Create an Appropriate Sleep Environment

In order to re-establish regular sleep patterns, it is important that your bed and bedroom become associated with sleep, not activities like watching television or writing letters. If you cannot get to sleep, or wake up, don't toss and turn, get up and do something and then go back to bed and try again. In addition, try to take your rest periods in an environment not associated with sleep, i.e. a chair or sofa, so that 'bed' starts to equate with sleep.

(4) Daytime Activity

Try not to sleep during the day; rest instead. Continue to gradually build up your daytime activity.

Finally, it does take time, sometimes weeks, to develop new habits, so don't be disappointed if they do not happen quickly. As long as you persevere, you will be able to establish a regular, refreshing sleep pattern.

Recommended Reading:

Trudie Chalder, *Coping With Chronic Fatigue*, Sheldon Press 1995, 2nd edition, Chapter 4, pages 41–51. ISBN 0-85969-685-5. Price: £5.99.

Why Healthy Eating?

When you are ill it is important to eat a balanced nutritious diet to give your body the best chance of recovery. In chronic fatigue syndrome this can be difficult because, due to tiredness, people find it difficult to prepare meals, which may result in a poor diet.

What Should I Eat?

- You should aim to eat three regular meals a day and avoid snacks in between.
- If you feel the need to eat between meals, try fruit or vegetables.
- Grill, bake, steam, casserole, poach, boil or microwave food instead of frying it.
- Use skimmed or semi-skimmed milk.
- Replace meat with fish, especially oily fish such as mackerel, salmon, tuna and herring.
- Use low-fat cheese or cottage cheese instead of high-fat hard cheeses like Stilton or Cheddar.
- Replace butter with a low-fat margarine.
- Use olive oil or rapeseed oil in cooking if needed.
- Choose foods labelled 'no added sugar' and cut down on processed foods.
- Drink unsweetened fruit juice or sugar-free drinks.
- Eat high-fibre foods such as pasta, rice, pitta bread, wholegrain breakfast cereals.

Most people with chronic fatigue syndrome find that alcohol makes them worse, as a result of sensitivity. The maximum safe weekly consumption of alcohol is 21 units for men and 14 units for women. One unit of alcohol is a half-pint of normal strength beer, lager or cider; or one measure of spirits; or one small glass of wine, sherry or liqueur. However, if you are on medication, especially amitriptyline, it is advisable not to drink alcohol, as the drug enhances the effects of alcohol.

What About Special Diets?

There is no evidence at present that 'special diets' help. There may be a few people who are intolerant of or allergic to certain foods but this does not always seem to be a reason for their tiredness. Some people find they have a *Candida* problem, and may try an anti-*Candida* diet, but again there is little evidence at present that this helps.

The important point is that you follow a healthy diet that is low in sugar and fat, and high in fibre, carbohydrates and proteins. If in doubt, ask to see a dietician.

What About Supplements?

There is some evidence that evening primrose oil can assist in some cases but this does not work for all. At present the evidence on the use and results obtained from supplements is limited. Some people say that they have benefited from taking different vitamins. If you would like to try a vitamin, choose a multi-vitamin and take only the recommended daily dose stated on the bottle or by the pharmacist.

Exercise?

Exercise is important to stop muscle wasting and to keep your joints mobile. It can also help you relax and sleep better. Like everything else in chronic fatigue syndrome it is important to pace yourself and take things gradually. Your body is like a partially charged battery with only so much charge for each day. It may not have enough 'charge' to cope with energetic exercise.

Don't forget you may already be doing some form of exercise such as walking to the bathroom, or stretching in bed.

When recovery is under way you may feel like becoming more active. It is important that exercise is started very gently and built up over time – don't leap back into things expecting to be like you were before you were ill. Like all other activities, exercise needs to be added in gradually in a step-wise systematic way. Walking is frequently chosen as an initial exercise. It is better to measure the time you walk rather than the distance or by counting steps.

The type of exercise will depend on you and your current level of ability; this will be discussed more fully in therapy sessions.

The type of exercise to start with might be:

- a 2–3 minute walk each day, or
- a flight of stairs, or
- going to the swimming pool once a week and paddling for five minutes.

The amount you do is then built up gradually over time, just as you would for any other daily activity. Exercise does not necessarily mean sport, especially in the early stages. *In time*, it may mean a return to playing a light game of football, cycling, walking or doing a keep-fit class. However, intense exercise using equipment or in a class should not be attempted until you are capable of performing high-energy daily activities, such as, climbing the stairs without fatigue or after effect.

Havering Hospitals NHS Trust: Booklet Number Five

Feelings and Thoughts

© CFS Team, Havering Hospitals NHS Trust, 1997
First produced by Diane Cox, 1994

> Adapted from an original idea by Dr Simon Hatcher
> Leeds Fatigue Clinic
> Seacroft Hospital, Leeds LS14 6UH

Chronic Fatigue Syndrome Diagnostic and Management Service
Essex Centre for Neurological Sciences
Oldchurch Hospital
Romford, Essex RM7 0BE

Feelings

Having feelings is part of being human. They are a normal part of daily life. Everybody has feelings, but sometimes the way we express our feelings can be very different. If we deny our true feelings this not only affects our psychological functioning but also quite often our physical functioning. This 'shutting off' could lead to problems such as anxiety or depression. Sometimes it is our life experience that affects the way we deal with our feelings. It may be that we learn throughout childhood that feelings are unacceptable or unimportant. How many people have been told to 'pull yourself together'; 'snap out of it'; 'grow up'? These comments teach us to suppress or put a lid on emotions.

This may continue into adulthood and we learn to suppress or deny feelings so that we do not have to experience extra pain if they are acknowledged. We may even be frightened of upsetting others if we do express our true feelings.

We have found that if one feeling is repressed then all feelings are 'dampened down' to a certain extent. Energy is therefore used trying to hold in emotion. Often, it can be helpful to find a person who can help you look at emotions such as sadness, guilt, loneliness, anger, isolation, boredom, depression and anxiety. Remember, though, people closest to you may also be dealing with their own emotions about your illness.

Thoughts, Feelings and Behaviour

With any long-term illness, it can be very difficult to retain a positive outlook in the face of prolonged disability, restriction of everyday life and absence of a ready cure. The feelings that can be associated with chronic fatigue syndrome such as frustration, anger, irritability, anxiety, demoralization and profound change in mood can impair recovery. Thoughts, feelings and actions interlink with one another: what we do influences thoughts and feelings and, equally, the way we think can affect actions and feelings. For example, thoughts like 'I won't be able to do this properly' make it hard to even start anything. Equally, you may find yourself feeling worried, frustrated or helpless before or during an activity. These feelings are often linked to thoughts that may be running through your mind at the time. For example, thoughts such as 'I can't imagine getting over this' or 'I might make myself worse' are likely to contribute to feelings of fearfulness or helplessness which are not only distressing but will hold you back.

These types of thoughts are common in prolonged illness, and because of the way they make people feel and their impact on behaviour they are known as 'negative thoughts'. Alternatively, thoughts such as 'I won't know whether I can get over this until I try', 'I don't know whether I will feel worse, and I might even feel better' are likely to make you feel optimistic and in control. In other words, a change in one area will often lead to a change in the others.

Characteristics of Negative Thoughts

Negative thoughts are often called *automatic*, because they tend to appear suddenly of their own accord, without any conscious or deliberate effort. They can be very difficult to switch off and often appear quite *logical and plausible*; it may not occur to you to question them, although if you do, you will probably find that they are not necessarily always accurate. There are often alternative ways of viewing things that will be more helpful and enable you to feel better and do more. Everyone will have experienced negative thoughts whether they are ill or not. It is important to remember that the negative thoughts have become more frequent as a consequence of your illness.

Overcoming Negative Thoughts

The first step in overcoming negative thoughts is identifying them. This can be difficult because of their habitual and automatic nature; with regular practice it will become easier. Once you can identify them easily, the next step involves examining and critically evaluating them and looking for more helpful alternatives.

(1) *Recording negative thoughts*. Keep an eye on your mood and when it changes for the worse, try to complete a self-assessment form. You may find that the same thoughts occur again and again. In particular, look

out for negative thoughts that occur before or during activity. Once identified, the next step is to evaluate the thoughts you identify and look for more helpful alternatives.

(2) *What is the evidence* for *and* against *what you are thinking?* When negative thoughts occur, they tend to either ignore facts, or select only the evidence which supports them. For example, if you have a negative thought like 'I will never get over this', you may find yourself remembering times when you've had setbacks, techniques that haven't worked and examples of other people who have had CFS for years. Don't just accept this; instead pause, and look at *all* the facts of the situation. Ask yourself whether all of these facts back up what you are thinking. If some evidence contradicts the negative thought then there is probably an alternative way of viewing the situation. For example, alternatives might include successes you have had, progress made so far, and examples of people who have successfully overcome CFS.

(3) *What errors are you making in your thinking?* One feature of negative thoughts is that they frequently involve distortions of reality. They may well involve errors such as:

(a) **All or nothing thinking, looking at things in black or white terms.**
Example: 'If I can't do this activity well I might as well not bother'.

(b) **Jumping to conclusions.**
Example: 'I couldn't manage that walk, I must be a complete failure'.

(c) **Catastrophizing; getting things out of proportion.**
Example: 'My muscles ache, that must mean I'm doing myself some permanent damage'.

(d) **Placing little emphasis on positive aspects.**
Example: 'Today was a terrible day, nothing went right, I've achieved nothing' or ' My life has been a complete waste because of this illness'.

(e) **Personalizing.**
Example: 'The illness is my fault'.

(f) **Overgeneralizing.**
Example: 'I tried reducing my rest before and it didn't work then, so it's not going to work now'.

These are just some examples of negative thoughts and thinking errors. If you can stand back from the thought and dissect it for these errors, it will be easier to come up with alternatives.

Use the Self-Assessment Forms to assist.

(4) *Advantages and disadvantages.* Ask yourself, does this style of thinking influence how you feel and what you do? What are the advantages and disadvantages of thinking this way? Is the way you are thinking now helping you achieve your goal, or is it standing in the way?

(5) *Thought switching.* Once you have been able to identify negative thoughts you may find that you have a constant recurring negative thought. A technique to change this thought to a positive thought is *thought switching*:
  (a) Write down the *negative thought:* 'I am never going to get better'.
  (b) Write down a *positive alternative thought:* 'I am going to get better'.
  (c) Think of the negative thought, say to yourself *switch*, think of the positive thought, then say *switch back*, and think of the negative thought, then *switch*, think of the positive thought. Do this a number of times, always ending with the positive thought.

Try to use the technique each time the original or a different recurring negative thought occurs.

(6) *Cognitive rehearsal.* If you identify a situation that increases anxiety or your negative thought patterns, for example, holding a conversation, visiting friends, think of the situation in your mind and play the whole scene through. Often when you rehearse a situation through like this in your mind before the event, it makes the actual event easier to manage.

Summary

It is extremely important to challenge negative thoughts systematically in order to overcome them. Writing them down is an effective way of doing this and allows you to be more objective. *Writing down alternatives gives you more power.*

Don't worry if you cannot come up with alternatives when you feel badly upset. Just write down the negative thoughts, distract yourself and then return to the task when you feel calmer. Try not to feel discouraged if the same thoughts recur again and again; this is quite likely to happen, as negative thinking is often well established. The more often it occurs the more chance you have to challenge it.

Havering Hospitals NHS Trust: Booklet Number Six

The Way Forward?

© CFS Team, Havering Hospitals NHS Trust, 1997
First produced by Diane Cox, 1994

> Adapted from an original idea by Dr Simon Hatcher
> Leeds Fatigue Clinic
> Seacroft Hospital, Leeds LS14 6UH

Chronic Fatigue Syndrome Diagnostic and Management Service
Essex Centre for Neurological Sciences
Oldchurch Hospital
Romford, Essex RM7 0BE

Illness and Other People

The key to coping with relationships in any chronic illness is *communication*. Being open about how you feel both physically and psychologically is important. Let people know how you feel and what you can and cannot do in a clear and consistent way. It is a lot harder for people to cope if they have to guess. It is also easier if you can give them some positive feedback for helpful things. Communication works both ways.

Living with someone who has chronic fatigue syndrome can be difficult. The partners or families of sufferers have to go through a type of grief reaction. They have to cope with someone who often looks 'normal' but who does not have the energy to do anything. It is like losing someone who has not actually gone – confusing and painful. It can also be frustrating to cope with changes in symptoms – for example, preparing to go out only to find you no longer have the energy.

Friends and family have to find some 'time for themselves'. They may think 'I shouldn't have needs because I'm not the one who is sick'. This is not true – it is just as important for them to meet their own needs. Another automatic thought that they may have is 'she's just doing it because she doesn't love me'. This is often paired with sufferers thinking 'I'm a burden and you're tolerating me to be nice'. It is easy to see how these thoughts can grow and feed on each other if there is poor communication.

Irritability

Irritability commonly occurs in chronic fatigue syndrome. It is unpleasant for the patient as well as the person on the receiving end. Often, the same things keep causing arguments. If you can, try to keep a record of arguments over a week and see if there is anything that consistently starts a quarrel. If there is, either find some way of avoiding it or try to talk it out when you are feeling reasonably well; arrange a time some days ahead to settle the matter.

Educating Others

It is important to inform people to help them understand your illness and that you are not 'making up' the symptoms. It is not your fault that you are ill any more than if you broke your leg or had a heart attack. Sharing literature can help others see that they are not alone in having to cope with the consequences of the illness.

Work

In many ways this is similar to dealing with other people at home. The golden rule is communication. Try to be honest with your boss. If possible, negotiate a change in hours. You may not be able to reduce your hours but if the time is flexible then you might be able to make travelling to work easier. Feeling guilty about 'letting the firm down' and 'not pulling my weight' is unavoidable. You may feel that your co-workers think you are lazy. Again, being open and honest about your illness is the best way of managing this. Remember: where possible, delegation is the best form of management!

If you are attempting to return to work in alternative employment, it is better to consider voluntary work first, so that you are able slowly to build up hours over time before returning to paid employment. The approach is the same as with all other activities, reintroduction over time.

Preparing for the Future

In order to maintain the gains you have made or will make, it is vital to ensure that the steps you have taken become part of everyday life. You will also need to make sure that you keep a sensible equilibrium, and that your days are balanced between different types of activity and relaxation. You should continue to work on targets and goals as you have been doing, systematically and gradually. You will probably find it useful and most helpful to continue to set yourself weekly targets, broken down into manageable chunks that are practised regularly. Keep a diary of any remaining tasks until you can achieve them consistently and regularly, without feeling excessively tired. Once you have *conquered* targets you need to make sure that they or their equivalent become part of your normal routine, i.e. do things regularly so things remain manageable, for example, supermarket shopping once a week. Once it is part of your routine, you will eventually be able do it without thinking about it and without effort.

Making Changes

Making changes is an important part of sustaining a lasting improvement. If you don't capitalize on your gains, you will find that they evaporate; this ties in with making sure that your targets become incorporated into your daily life. If you have been working on walking a certain amount every day, talking to people for increasing amounts of time, and carrying out tasks requiring concentration, one way of bringing all these together (if you are ready for it) is to start going back to work or doing a voluntary job. The important factor is to maintain the same structure and amount of activity each day to reduce the chances of returning to the CFS pattern of peaks and troughs: switching between doing too much and too little.

If you have been ill for a long time, you may have lost some of the things you had when you were last well. If this is the case, then making changes involves a fair amount of rebuilding, and doing things that you may not have done for a long time. Readjusting to a normal life can be a difficult and even an alarming prospect, but feeling apprehensive does not mean that you are going to fail, it simply means that you are moving into the final stages of recovery. If you have come this far, there is no reason why you should not overcome the final hurdles.

The important thing is to remember to take things gradually. If something seems unmanageable, break it down. Second, don't be critical of yourself if you feel apprehensive; this is a perfectly normal and understandable reaction. However, keep an eye on your negative thoughts that may creep in, as apprehension and anxiety can breed unhelpful thinking patterns. If you find yourself thinking that you cannot do it, it's too much, there's no point, you'll fail, etc., then remind yourself that there are other, more useful ways of viewing the situation; get out your negative thoughts diary or self-assessment forms and look for alternatives.

Avoid Old Patterns

You need to beware of returning to doing exactly what you were doing before the illness, as this could involve picking up old behaviour patterns which may have made you vulnerable to the illness in the first place. This is particularly apt if you used to live your life at a very fast pace, or if you had extremely high expectations of yourself and how you should perform. Take the fact that you have had chronic fatigue syndrome as a cue for moderating the pace of things.

Coping with Setbacks

As you may have already found, recovery from CFS can involve the odd setback from time to time. You may have had setbacks during your treatment – periods when all the symptoms and tiredness seem to overwhelm you again, everything goes wrong and you wonder whether there's any point in going on. It is absolutely normal to have these setbacks, which are simply stages on the way to recovery. If a setback happens it does not mean you are relapsing; it is simply an unpleasant but temporary state of affairs that can be overcome.

There are some important guidelines to follow if you have a setback:

(1) *Don't panic:* remember that setbacks are not a disaster. As long as you don't give up you can overcome them.

(2) *Make use of setbacks:* you can learn from them, as they teach you about the sorts of things that make you feel worse, and give you a chance to practise and strengthen what you have learnt.

(3) *Setbacks do not mean treatment has not worked or is not working.* Look at what is causing you problems, look at the pattern of activity and symptoms and plan your programme accordingly, i.e. as before, planned, manageable, regular and frequent rest and activity blocks.

(4) *Remember the improvements you have made:* even if they seem to have gone at the moment, they will come back; follow point 3 and you can ensure they return.

(5) *Don't feel that you have to start again from scratch:* the more you have improved the worse your setback can seem in contrast. Seeing it as starting from scratch will just make you feel worse. It is highly unlikely that it will take as long before you are back to the level you were at before your setback.

(6) *Don't blame yourself:* setbacks can happen, and the best way of looking at them is as a problem to be solved, not as a rod with which to beat yourself.

(7) *Keep trying!* even if you can't get over a setback immediately, don't give up. You will overcome it, given time and perseverance.

The best way of beating setbacks is to be aware that they may happen, and plan for them. There are specific circumstances that increase the risk of a setback: severe physical illness; stressful life events; changing jobs; bereavement; moving house. At times you may also find yourself slipping back if you simply stop using the techniques used in treatment, if you plunge headlong into a frantic burst of activity or, conversely, if you retreat into inactivity. This can be avoided if you stick by the principles of consistency, grading, pacing and moderation.

(Acknowledgement is made to the work of Professor Simon Wessely and colleagues, King's College Hospital, London, for the above suggestions.)

Finally, don't let being a 'CFS' or 'ME' patient become your sole identity. Value yourself for who you are rather than what you can and cannot do.

Suggested Further Reading

Trudie Chalder, *Coping With Chronic Fatigue*, Sheldon Press, 1995, 2nd edition. ISBN 0-85969-685-5.Price: £5.99.

Appendix 2
Selected Information Sheets

Information Sheet 5:
Occupational Therapy and Lifestyle Management

Occupational therapists (OTs) work towards maximizing levels of independence and ability. This means working with you in deciding whether changes are needed in your lifestyle. This includes talking through your current abilities, routines and ways of coping.

Your OT will discuss your current lifestyle with you. You will then be offered the opportunity to look at ways of making adjustments so that, in time, you are able to do more for yourself. To do this, we concentrate on how your thoughts, feelings and behaviour interact with each other and the possible need to make changes in order to move you forwards.

During your stay, you will be assessed by one of our specialist OTs. You will then be given an individual therapeutic programme. The programme is tailored to each individual's need and taken at each person's pace. This may mean that information given to you is covered at a different speed to that provided to your neighbours on the ward. You will be seen regularly during your admission to continue working on your programme and to address any difficulties.

You will be guided through a set of booklets which discuss various aspects of lifestyle management. You may also be asked to complete some short written exercises regarding the structure of your day, current levels of ability and future plans.

We aim to help you gain a better understanding of your illness and how to cope with it. You can begin to implement some of the ideas for yourself whilst on the ward. As you gain more knowledge, and with the continued support and guidance of your therapist, you can learn how to adapt the programme to your home situation.

Lifestyle management education does not represent a 'cure' for chronic fatigue syndrome. Neither is it prescriptive or inflexible. It is designed to help you learn methods of coping with your illness, to feel more in control of the symptoms and to increase your potential for recovery.

Information Sheet 11:
Guidance for Family and Friends

From experience, we have found that patients respond better to their treatment programme if visiting is restricted during the first few weeks of their stay. This will allow the various investigations and therapeutic interventions to be carried out with the minimum of disturbance to the patient, staff and other patients on the ward.

We would therefore request that the patient receives no visitors during the first two weeks and that, after this time, visiting hours be negotiated with the occupational therapist responsible for his/her care.

On admission, patients are assessed and entered into a therapeutic programme. You will be given a contact name and telephone number to find out how your relative or friend is progressing whilst on the ward and to answer any queries.

After discharge, patients are followed up, either in the outpatient clinic or by a review admission. Ongoing support and advice are available from CFS team therapists and the National ME Centre, based at Harold Wood Hospital.

On returning home, people often need time and space to implement some of the changes they have learnt whilst in hospital. It is important to remember that recovery takes patience and persistence.

Information Sheet 12:
What to Expect on Discharge

On discharge, it is anticipated that you will have an understanding of your individual programme and how to progress it. Opportunities to discuss future plans are integrated into your sessions with the therapists and time can be allocated for your relatives to ask questions, if required.

Basically, we would suggest that you continue with your programme at home and work towards your own goals and aims, as discussed with the therapists.

Once at home, it is important to maintain positive changes and to avoid slipping back into any potentially negative patterns.

It is also important to emphasize that not everyone leaves hospital with the changes they had anticipated! Whilst people can make improvements on the ward, it is often necessary to take a step backwards before going forwards. People may find that they need time at home to begin to put the lifestyle management techniques into practice.

Future Follow Up and Contact

Prior to discharge, the therapists will discuss follow-up arrangements with you. There are options for follow up and the team will help you decide which is the most suitable for you. You may be offered an outpatient appointment to attend clinic, usually in 4–6 months' time. You may be offered a further inpatient stay (subject to referring Health Authority approval). If this is the case, your next stay will usually be between five and 14 days in duration.

Before you leave the ward, nursing staff will try to let you know the date and time of your next follow-up medical clinic appointment. However, if this is not possible, your follow-up details will be sent to you in the post shortly after discharge.

Ongoing support and advice is available from the therapists by either letter or telephone contact. Occasionally, it may be necessary to arrange an additional outpatient appointment with one of the therapists. If this is the case, it will be arranged between you and the therapist concerned. Further support is available via letter and telephone contact with the National ME Centre at Harold Wood Hospital.

Remember: it takes time to recover! Give yourself time and space to try out the techniques you have learnt in hospital. Recognize any changes you need to make and the successes you achieve.

Appendix 3: Useful Addresses

Occupational Therapy Organizations

The College of Occupational Therapists
106–114 Borough High Street
London SE1 1LB
UK
Tel: 0171 450 2329
Fax: 0171 450 2299
Website: http://www.cot.co.uk/

The Canadian Association of Occupational Therapists
Carleton Technology and Training Centre
Suite 3400 Carleton University Campus
1125 Colonel By Drive
Ottawa K15 5R1
Canada
Tel: 613 523 2268
Fax: 613 523 2552
Website: http://www.caot.ca/

CFS/ME Organizations

American Association for Chronic Fatigue Syndrome
c/o Harborview Medical Center
325 9th Avenue, Box 359780
Seattle, Washington State
USA 98104
Website: http://www.aacfs.org/
A non-profit organization of research scientists, physicians, licensed medical healthcare professionals, and other individuals and institutions interested in promoting the stimulation, coordination, and exchange of

ideas for CFS research and patient care, as well as periodic reviews of current clinical, research and treatment ideas on CFS for the benefit of CFS patients and others.

Doctor NET online – Chronic Fatigue Resources
Website: http://www.comedserv.com/fatigue.htm

Website with access to a number of electronic resources linked to CFS/ME.

Support Groups

UK

The National ME Centre
DSC
Harold Wood Hospital
Romford, Essex RM3 0BE
UK
Tel: 01708 378050
Fax: 01708 378032
Email: nmecent@ac.aol.com
A registered charity that supports patients and professionals with verbal and written information on CFS/ME. The centre runs support and medical clinics for advice on management for those who already have a confirmed diagnosis. The centre is committed to the education of all healthcare professionals involved in CFS/ME care and management and has held two international conferences, one in 1996 for GPs in particular and one in 1999 for all healthcare professionals.

Westcare (reg. Charity No. 900619)
155 Whiteladies Road
Clifton, Bristol BS8 2RF
UK
Tel: 0117 9239341
Fax: 0117 9239347
A registered charity set up in 1989 to provide services and support for people with PVFS/ME/CFS. Its main service is a clinic in Bristol that provides consultations with professional advisors and counsellors.

ME Association
4 Corringham Road
Stanford le Hope, Essex SS17 0AH, UK
Tel: 01375 642466
Website: http://www.compulink.co.uk/~deepings/
A registered charity which aims to support all those affected by ME by providing specialist information and advice services, literature and self-help groups. It also promotes research into causes and effects of the illness; increases public awareness of ME; provides training for health and other professionals; raises funds for research; and campaigns for appropriate high-quality services for sufferers.

ME Association Young People's Group*
PO Box 81
Evesham, Worcestershire WR11 5WB, UK
Email: meaypg@cix.compulink.co.uk
Website: http://www.cix.co.uk/~meaypg/index.htm
*This group is associated with the ME Association

Action for ME
PO Box 1302
Wells, Somerset BA5 1YE, UK
24-hour hotline: 0891 122976
Young Action Online
Email: jane@jafc.demon.co.uk
Website: http://www.afme.org.uk/
A UK-based national membership organization and registered charity. Its aims are to campaign for more recognition, research and better care and benefits for ME sufferers, and to provide information, self-help and support services to people with ME, their carers, family and friends.

USA

The CFIDS Association of America
PO Box 220398
Charlotte, North Carolina
USA 28222-0398
Voice Messages: 800/442-3437
Fax: 704/365-9755
Website: http//www.cifds.org/
A national charitable organization dedicated to the care of CFS/ME. It has been running since 1987 and has been actively involved in education about CFS/ME.

Canada

The ME Association of Canada
Suite 200, 246 Queen Street
Ottawa, Ontario
Canada K1P 5E4
Tel: 613 563-1565
Fax: 613 567-0614
Email: infor@mecan.ca
Website: http://www.mecan.ca
A national association founded in 1987, which provides referrals to area support groups, legal assistance on such matters as disability pension and tax claims, medical literature and counselling.

Australia

ME/CFS Society (S.A) Inc.
GPO Box 383
Adelaide
South Australia 5001
Australia
Tel: 08 8373 3379; Counselling: 08 8266 5833 (10:00 am–4:00 pm, local time)
Website: http://www.span.com.au/me/
At the above website addresses are available for groups in New South Wales, Australian Capital Territory, Queensland, Victoria and Western Australia.

Glossary

Advantages and disadvantages is a technique used to challenge dysfunctional thoughts. The person considers the advantage of the particular thought and then the disadvantages, to assist in reaching a resolution or a change in thought pattern.

Alternative thoughts is a technique used to challenge dysfunctional thoughts; in particular, recurring negative automatic thoughts. The person is asked to consider alternative reasons why something may have happened.

Arbitrary inference is a thinking style where the person has a tendency to jump to conclusions.

Attribution is a person's individual perception of fact.

Beliefs are what a person feels is real and true, something on which they base their trust and confidence.

Chronic fatigue syndrome (CFS) is a new onset of persistent or relapsing, debilitating fatigue or easy fatigability in a person who has no previous history of similar symptoms, that has lasted longer than six months, is disabling and affects physical and mental functioning.

Cognitive behaviour therapy (CBT) is an approach that integrates cognitive and behavioural treatment principles. The person is helped by the therapist to recognize, evaluate and modify patterns of distorted thinking and dysfunctional behaviour. CBT is therefore based on the theory that inaccurate unhelpful beliefs, ineffective coping behaviour, negative mood states, social problems and pathophysiological processes all interact to perpetuate illness.

Cognitive deficiency is a thinking style whereby the person has a tendency to disregard an important aspect of a life situation, and ignore or fail to integrate or utilize relevant information derived from experience (learning from past experience).

Cognitive rehearsal is a technique used to change dysfunctional thoughts, or reduce anxiety about a situation. The event is played out or 'rehearsed' in the person's mind. Another view is to think of this technique as mental role play.

Dichotomous thinking is a thinking style whereby the person tends to evaluate events in extreme terms with no attention being paid to the 'middle ground'. They tend to think in 'black and white' terms.

Dysfunctional thoughts are thoughts that hinder, work against or limit a person achieving, and can relate to any aspect of daily life.

Evidence for and against is a technique used to challenge and change dysfunctional thoughts. The person is asked to consider the evidence he/she has for the thought pattern and the evidence against the thoughts, i.e. testing the belief based on available evidence.

'Friend' technique is a technique used to challenge and change dysfunctional thoughts. In essence you would say to the person, 'would you say this to a friend?', i.e. consider how you would react if a friend told you what you have just said and then consider how you would respond.

Inference chains follows an 'if A then B' form of reasoning, i.e. thoughts that follow a sequence. In other words, the person associates one idea or outcome with another. Usually the subsequent inference is more global and emotionally laden.

Magnification (or minimization) is a thinking style whereby the person has a tendency to exaggerate the importance of a negative event (or to undervalue the importance of a positive one).

Negative automatic thoughts (NATs) are a type of thought pattern. As the name implies, the thoughts tend to always be of a negative nature and automatically come to mind. They are usually the immediate consciously available thoughts.

Over-generalization is a thinking style whereby the person has a tendency to derive global conclusions on the basis of little evidence or a single event.

Personalization is a thinking style whereby the person has a tendency to relate external events to him/herself when there is no basis for making such a connection.

Randomized controlled trials (RCTs) are experimental trials wherein subjects are randomly allocated into groups to limit bias through selection. One group will receive treatment and the other will receive no active treatment and is generally termed the 'control' group.

Rules are a person's operating instructions for life. In general they relate to instructions and beliefs that enable happiness and avoid pain and unpleasantness, for example 'I must be approved of at all times' or 'I must always put the needs of others first'.

Thought switching/stopping is a technique used to assist the person in changing or ceasing the recurring negative automatic thought. The person is encouraged to think of a prepared positive alternate thought to the one he/she has most regularly, and every time the negative thought occurs to switch to thinking of the positive one instead, or to say 'stop' to him/herself to stop the thought.

Index